"A riveting insight into the act of survival. This book will break your heart right open, and that's a good thing—vulnerability draws us closer."

Mike Downie, filmmaker and Co-Founder of the Gord Downie & Chanie Wenjack Fund.

•

"The personal stories in this book all begin at the moment when our normal routines are swept away by illness, trauma, or death. The ensuing transformations prove that mortality is a great teacher. A brave and compelling collection."

Robert Everett-Green is a Toronto journalist and author of the novel *In A Wi e Country*.

•

"This brave collection speaks to our common humanity, to the devastating losses we experience by being alive. It's what results when big questions, vital questions, are let loose in the world. These shared stories resonate with deep feeling, wisdom, and courage."

Camilla Gibb is an award-winning author of four novels, and most recently, a memoir, *This Is Happy*.

•

"A deeply moving mosaic of lives lived and lost, generously shared, that touches the soul. There is rawness here—of pain, grief, joy, and transformed lives."

Mary Jo Haddad CM, LLD (Hon), RN, former President and CEO, The Hospital for Sick Children, and Chancellor, University of Windsor.

•

"These stories of survival and triumph come out of intense pain, loss, and sadness. The effect can be initially shattering, then affirming, and at times exhilarating. I applaud the courage of these storytellers."

Chaviva Hošek, OC, Professor at Munk School of Global Affairs & Public Policy and former CEO of the Canadian Institute for Advanced Research.

•

"A searing, compelling examination of how individuals process and ultimately survive trauma, pain, and loss. This emotionally honest book is simultaneously brutal, beautiful and deeply inspiring."

Jennifer Meeropol, grand-daughter of Ethel and Julius Rosenberg, and Executive Director of the Rosenberg Fund For Children in Easthampton, Massachusetts (www.rfc.org).

# A

Personal stories

# PERFECT

of trauma and

# OFFERING

transformation

# A

Personal stories

# PERFECT

of trauma and

# OFFERING

transformation

Edited by
Harold Heft, Suzanne Heft, Peter O'Brien

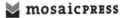

**Library and Archives Canada Cataloguing in Publication**

Title: A Perfect Offering: Personal stories of trauma and transformation / edited by Harold Heft, Suzanne Heft and Peter O'Brien.
Other titles: Perfect offering (2020) | Personal stories of trauma and transformation

Names: Heft, Harold, 1964-2015, editor. | Heft, Suzanne, 1967- editor. | O'Brien, Peter, 1957- editor.

Description: Essays.

Identifiers: Canadiana (print) 20200287036 | Canadiana (ebook) 20200287494 | ISBN 9781771615129 (softcover) | ISBN 9781771615136 (PDF) | ISBN 9781771615143 (HTML) | ISBN 9781771615150 (Kindle)

Subjects: LCSH: Psychic trauma. | LCSH: Canadian essays—21st century. | CSH: Canadian essays (English)—21st century.

Classification: LCC PS8367.T7 P47 2020 | DDC C814/.06080353—dc23

Published by Mosaic Press, Oakville, Ontario, Canada, 2020.

MOSAIC PRESS, Publishers

Printed and bound in Canada.

Designed by Andrea Tempesta • www.flickr.com/photos/andreatempesta

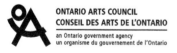

ONTARIO ARTS COUNCIL
CONSEIL DES ARTS DE L'ONTARIO
an Ontario government agency
un organisme du gouvernement de l'Ontario

Funded by the Government of Canada
Financé par le gouvernement du Canada | Canada

We acknowledge the Ontario Arts Council
for their support of our publishing program

**MOSAIC PRESS**
1252 Speers Road, Units 1 & 2, Oakville, Ontario, L6L 5N9
(905) 825-2130 • info@mosaic-press.com • www.mosaic-press.com

For Harold,

the beginning and the completion of this project.

And for Sam and John.

# Contents

---

Introduction                                                                    10

Harold Heft—*The World I Once Inhabited: Draft One*                              14
Andrea Aster—*Jack*                                                             20
Jennifer Finney Boylan—*How to Save Your Own Life*                              26
Jennifer Boyle—*Unremembered*                                                   34
Steve Brearton—*Invisible Tracks*                                              44
Aimee Bruner and Mishi Methven—*We Eat Ice Cream for Breakfast*                 52
Janet Culliton—*Grace Notes*                                                    58
Vicki Dunleavy—*All the Other Kids Died*                                        64
Janelle A. Girard—*Walking as I Wake*                                          72
Lynn Gluckman—*To My 17-Year-Old Self*                                          80
Trevor Greene—*A Long, Bleak Christmas*                                         88
Teva Harrison—*Still Here*                                                     94
Judith John—*Brain Drain. Brain Trust.*                                        100
Jules Arita Koostachin—*Intertwined: Speaking Our Truths*                       108
Alison Langham—*The Old Me, The New Me*                                        118
Valerie McDonald—*No One Said the D-Word*                                       126
Rocky Morra—*My Sister Tina, the Strong One*                                    134
Marina Nemat—*The Chemistry Notebook*                                          140
Peter O'Brien—*Walking Shadows*                                                148
Eric Petersiel—*"Daddy, what's this?"*                                         154
Ed Pien—*The Tangled Garden*                                                   162
Neena Saloya—*Navigating My Darkness*                                           170
Ellen Schwartz—*The Miracle of Jacob*                                          176
Kenneth Sherman—*Poems from Jogging with the Great Ray Charles*                 182
charles c. smith—*waiting to explode: four poems*                              190
Rabbi Yael Splansky—*Sermon for the Second Day of Rosh Hashanah*                198
Michelle Sylliboy—*A Song Dreams Within*                                        206
Andrea Warnick—*Honouring Aunt Catherine, and Beyond*                          216
Paul Watson—*Children*                                                         224
Alyssa Wooster—*It's Okay To Not Be Okay*                                       238
Bänoo Zan—*The Mirror Soliloquy*                                               244

Acknowledgements                                                               251

# Introduction

—

In his song "Anthem," Leonard Cohen writes:

> Forget your perfect offering
> There is a crack
> A crack in everything
> That's how the light gets in

In January 2014, at the age of 49, my husband Harold collapsed at work. He was subsequently diagnosed with an inoperable brain tumour, the same kind that took the life of Canadian musician Gord Downie of the Tragically Hip, and U.S. Senator John McCain. With brave determination, he submitted to all the medical intervention that was available, but less than two years later Harold slipped out of this world and into the next.

The idea for this book came from questions Harold turned over and over in his mind, obsessively, while he was ill. How do we human beings survive the traumas of our lives? What does the trauma take away from us? What is left behind?

In the summer of 2014, Harold and Peter sat outside in our garden with a warm sun slowly wandering back and forth among the stationary trees—and talked about beginnings and endings.

A talker all his life, and a writer by trade, Harold now struggled with words. His tumour affected the part of the brain that drives all communication. Through garbled syntax and fractured sentences unravelling in fits and starts, Harold spoke about his cancer:

"... I don't have any words! ..." he said. "I'm 49 ... my kids ... what about them? ... Pete, how old was your Dad when he died? ..."

"49," said Peter. "Never made it to 50. And then my mom was a widow with 10 kids, in New York, not her home city. I wasn't even two years old when he died."

The three of us starting talking about people we knew—family, friends, and colleagues—and how every single one of them had experienced some form of personal trauma in their own life or in the lives of the people closest to them. A young child who had died. Parents who had been killed in a car crash. A disease ravaging a body. A mind unravelling from the horrors of war.

This is not just the stuff of therapy and support groups. Certainly we live in a more confessional age than a few decades ago, but there is still stigma around various types of trauma, including sexual violence, mental illness, and systemic racism. In Western culture, we cling to our fear of death and we live without the public vocabulary to address those who grieve in our midst. Trauma is so much a part of our personal histories, each of us. G. K. Chesterton says: "We are all in the same boat, in a stormy sea, and we owe each other a terrible loyalty."

Over the coming weeks Harold and Peter envisioned a collection of these personal stories, written by the people they knew, and some they did not. They hoped that such a collection would give the contributors an opportunity—however partial, inadequate—to share their stories in whatever way they thought most appropriate. Harold hoped that a wider audience might find these stories enlightening, instructive or sympathetic, perhaps even comforting. After all, adversity often carries with it a profound feeling of isolation and loneliness—it's our common humanity, pulsing beneath the surface of everyday life.

Trauma divides us into "before" and "after." As Harold said in a moment of frustration and lucidity: "I was that person ... until suddenly, I was *not* that person."

There is no going back.

Each of us—children are particularly good at this—live our lives ignorant of the personal and collective storms that swirl around us: the tragedy and destruction on distant shores, the undiscovered country of our immediate neighbours. And then one day the storm is upon us—we witness trauma in our own lives and the lives of those we care about.

These forced awakenings can provide instructive lessons. In sharing them, we glimpse not just the ways in which humans endure, but also how we transform ourselves and each other.

Harold also began wondering, in words that began to arrange themselves on a page, about his own forced awakening. He was no longer able to write or type. Months had passed since he had been able to read Wallace Stevens or *The New Yorker*. He dictated emails and notes, and put me to work as his scribe:

– How do we define a life worth living?

– Is the worth related to endurance, experience, and achievement?

– Is it about overcoming challenges or enjoying our fleeting moments of joy?

– How do we journey from one day to the next with the understanding that inevitably death will occur?

– Why do we persist, as we listen to our breath and our heartbeat counting off the diminishing moments?

Harold's large, impossible questions.

In response, most of us only have small, inadequate answers.

In the months after Harold died, on 23 July 2015, I was numb. I was searching for meaning of my own. Pete and I haltingly began to pick up the pieces of this book. The two of us began to reconnect with potential contributors, some of whom had already handed in finished pieces. We started to edit, and to spread the word wider, inviting additional contributors. The pieces came pouring in.

This is the collection we have assembled. We are honoured to share them. Many are tough, emotional, wrenching. Each is a testament to the innate power in each human being to survive, and despite all odds, to tell the tale.

Sometimes only just.

There are stories here of the death of children, of living with chronic pain and disease, and military battle, of surviving sexual assault, terrorist attacks, imprisonment and torture, of giving birth to a new gender, of surviving the legacy of Canada's residential schools. In each story there is courage, dignity, proof of persistence.

Pete and I went back to Harold's notes for his own contribution to this book. His unfinished words. We decided to publish them as we found them. An imperfect offering, for sure.

One of the things grieving persons frequently do is wonder about what the dead person would have said or thought about some subject. As Pete and I edited this book of stories, I wondered what Harold would make of its final form.

In Japan, *Kintsukuroi* is the centuries-old art of fixing broken pottery. Rather than re-join ceramic pieces with a camouflaged adhesive, the technique employs a special tree sap lacquer dusted with powdered gold, silver, or platinum. Once completed, the seams glint within the visible cracks of the "repaired" piece. There is dignity and beauty in the imperfections. Rather than hiding or disguising the cracks, they are given their own life.

New cracks of light.

**Suzanne Heft**

Harold

# The World
# I Once Inhabited:
# Draft One

Heft

*[Over the last year of his life Harold was working on this book: talking and thinking about why it was needed, and contacting potential contributors. In his last months he started to make notes for his own contribution. By then his aphasia had worsened: he had trouble speaking and he couldn't type, read, or write. He dictated these words—in fits and starts—to his wife Suzanne. Interested in the craft of writing and a stickler for the right word in the right place, Harold would have redrafted this until he was satisfied, but he did not have that opportunity. The poem quoted toward the end of this piece is from Harold's book on the events surrounding the death of Montreal painter Alexander Bercovitch. The title of Harold's book on Bercovitch is* The Shape of this Dying.*]*

When I was 10 years old, I had open-heart surgery to repair a blockage in my aorta, leaving a foot-long scar stretching around my ribs to my back from where I was cut open. At the time, I knew it was dire and later understood that I could have easily died. Having dodged that bullet, as a grown man, I thought I was safe, at least for many decades.

In early 2014, without warning, I collapsed at work and was rushed to St. Michael's Hospital in Toronto where it was discovered that I had had a seizure. I later learned the seizure was the result of an inoperable brain tumour. I was 49 years old and the father of two young children, and suddenly I had to deal with the reality that this cancerous tumour would take my life at some point. The old life I knew fed that reality. The tumour would dictate every aspect of my existence forevermore.

One of my doctors points out: "everyone lives knowing that the end can come at any time." The difference with me, he says, is that I know what's coming. And living with that knowledge changes the nature of living itself.

So the question becomes, how do any of us live with this knowledge, or do we just choose not to think about it, until the very end comes?

Before I was diagnosed with brain cancer, I never thought about these matters. That might have been a good thing. Now I have no choice but to think about them—and that fundamentally changes the way I live my days.

Here is what life looks like for me now. There are many things that give me pleasure that I didn't necessarily think about before, including time spent with my children and family, a volunteer commitment, and spending more time with friends. However, I do grieve the lost opportunity to contribute to the world through my professional life. And I wonder what opportunities I am missing out on because I am not able to participate in the world I once inhabited.

The brain tumour took away the life I once led. It also places a giant question mark in front of the life before me. I cannot help but wonder what might have lay ahead.

Here are some questions that I now ask of myself and of the people around me:

How does my awareness of mortality change
the way I interact with the world?

Is it possible to live a full life with the knowledge that
death may come at any time, or is it necessary to do
so? Should I have been doing that all along?

At one point is it okay to say: "I have had a full
and good life and 'it's enough'?"

Who decides? And when?

What is a definition of a life well-lived under these
circumstances? How does time dictate this experience?

How has the tumour changed me?

It what way am still the person I always was?

These are some of the questions that I live with every day. I didn't spend much time with these questions before I was diagnosed with a brain tumour, and now they are with me all the time.

I have come to appreciate that many people—most of us—have to grapple with some form of adversity, whether physical, spiritual or psychological. I didn't give this much thought before. But almost everyone's life contains within it massive challenges of some sort, and often those challenges define who we are, whether we know it or not.

The most important lesson this illness has taught me—that I would not have otherwise understood—is that there is an abundance of goodness in people. Almost everyone has responded to me, and my family, with extraordinary generosity, compassion and kindness. Meals have been prepared and sent, my kids have been tirelessly car-pooled, neighbours have shovelled snow and rides have been provided to and from the hospital. An endless parade of small, good deeds that have lifted our spirits and helped us survive horror. I would never have known such goodness existed were it not for this experience.

But there is a flip side of course. I think about my family and what is going the happen to them.

I have spent time on matters of a practical nature: directives about financial matters, safe-guarding my children's educational future and so on. I have also thought about life-cycle events and milestones, the ones they will mark without me, and how I wish—how I hope—to be remembered. I have given instruction for the purchase of gifts for those occasions. I have enumerated and described to my wife trips I hope she will take with my sons, adventures I had that I hope they will have. Even as I offer these instructions, even as she agrees, we both silently acknowledge "the world has changed."

Sometimes a holiday is not a holiday, it is a pilgrimage.

Sometimes a new watch for the future bar mitzvah boy is not a time-piece but a talisman.

I once wrote in a poem, about an artist, a painter, and this line:

The immortality we seek
is in that which we take,

not in what we leave behind. It is
in the debt for marble chipped away,
not in the value

of the remaining statue.

The truth is I have lived a full and rich life for 50 years and if my life could be viewed as a statue, I would like to think it is a good one—honourable and dignified and meaningful.

My story did not end at the age of ten. Many more chapters and pages were still written. I am glad for that fact, and I acknowledge it each day that I still am able.

Everything is arbitrary and this is where my story ends.

————

**Harold Heft** believed in a story's fundamental power to illuminate life, to help us understand each other, and to bind human beings to each other. He published three books, including *The Shape of This Dying: Remembering Alexander Bercovitch* (Mosaic) and *Build a Better Book Club* (Macmillan Canada, written with Peter O'Brien). His articles and reviews appeared in *The Globe and Mail*, *National Post*, *The Jewish Daily Forward*, *Montreal Gazette* and *Tablet*. He graduated from McGill University, earned a PhD in literature from the University of Western Ontario, and was a visiting fellow at The Hebrew University of Jerusalem. He worked as a strategist and marketing communications executive at the University of Toronto, where he met Suzanne, and at The Hospital for Sick Children, and other charities. At age 51, after a diagnosis of an inoperable brain tumour, Harold died on 23 July 2015.

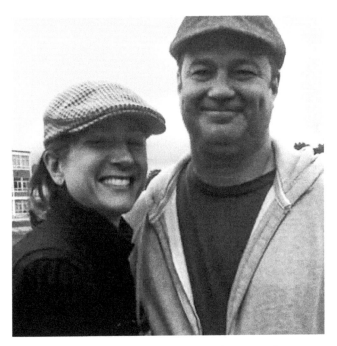
Suzanne and Harold Heft, October 2011, Toronto

Andrea

Jack

Aster

My son Jack died of a viral infection, four days after his first birthday. The chief paediatrician at the children's hospital pronounced him dead by telling us it was a "massive insult to the little fellow," such a gallant euphemism.

The night he died I learned a hospital's darkest secrets. When there's no hope left for your child, you get a whole empty ward to yourself. There are beds here for 20 little dead babies but yours is the only one, all hooked up to a monitor tuned to a dead channel. It's just a theatre for the living, really, a chance to say goodbye.

The hospital knows what you'd never think to pack, in your haste to accompany your dying child in the ambulance, the child you found five minutes after you put him peacefully to bed, now lying on his side and breathing as if sucking a milkshake from a straw, silhouette-shaped blood-stain on his crib sheet seeping from his nose, smell of shit. They have breast pumps on hand because you're still an engorged, nursing mom. Such a terrible thing; your body remains hopeful.

You lose 15 pounds in three days. The hell of sudden traumatic loss demands you hand over your flesh, your faith.

So, how does one survive?

First you find a place to cry. You cry endlessly. My tears were necessary as breath. I cried on the subway. It surprised me that my first instinct was a need to have strangers bear witness to my suffering. I didn't want anyone to actually engage me. I just needed to be seen as someone who truly couldn't walk credibly among the living. The code of the subway allows for all but the violent to do their thing unhindered. Years later, my husband Charles told me he cried on the subway too on his commute home—my private, guarded, formal, criminal-lawyer husband—he cried too.

The dissonance between my unblemished exterior and my shattered interior felt like an outrageous cosmic lie and awakened a proselytizing impulse within me. Though I didn't stride the aisles of the subway with blazing eyes and a sandwich board, my eyes spoke: listen up, a warning to all ye innocents who plan their futures and march blithely towards them. Guess what? This can happen. You too may fall down this well. Shred your hands on the clammy stone, then yield with dignity; trust me, there's no way out.

In my voracious post-trauma reading, when the only palatable text in the child-loss canon was the miserably named, *When the Bough Breaks*, I hit on a theory about why I cried on the subway instead of in bed. I read that, in Victorian times, black mourning clothes provided an outward display of a family's inner feelings. The clothes did the work of explaining one's pain to the community and soliciting its support, in a pre-vaccination age when kids died, a lot. One was advised to wear mourning clothes up to four years when your spouse died. It wasn't reassuring to read that a mother is to wear them "for as long as she felt so disposed," so deep is the pain.

When my subway journeys showed that the world at large wasn't going to give me a group hug, I decided to manage the pain by consulting a healer. Jeanette had thick copper hair to her waist, a pert nose and slightly pointy ears. It was rumoured she was of Druid descent and had mystical powers. I'll give her this: she did give off heat. "Everyone says that about me; take as much of it as you need," she said. She didn't have credentials, per se, but a friend I respected said Jeanette cured her lymphoma.

Jeanette wrote her prescriptions on unlined loose-leaf in faint ballpoint. There was a Delphic quality to her, her throaty voice cast at a pitch that invited a huge lean-in to catch the oracular pronouncements. She tilted her ear skyward as if receiving some exclusive frequency. There were many pauses. She channeled rather than spoke.

I was to drink only boiled water and eat only greens, certain grains and legumes—along with Mason-jar quantities of turmeric, cumin, and coriander. In our first session she cradled my skull in her hands for an hour and let the pain seep away. Vulnerable people go for stuff like this. I lasted three sessions.

I guess the key to my survival came as a revelation that had been there all along, hidden by the acuity of my suffering. When I walked out the hospital's emergency exit at dawn, leaving Charles behind to make funeral arrangements, I felt the absence of my boy in my arms for the first time. "I couldn't survive the death of my child," so many parents told me, in woeful stabs at empathy. Well, there I was, experiencing it for the first time, cut loose, with the novel feeling of weightlessness you'd imagine, after holding your babe to your body for a year.

So, here's the secret you can't anticipate. Sure, it's every parent's worst nightmare but it's also every parent's highest wish—*I'll never have to worry about him again.* Such a terrible revelation, such perverse freedom.

I'd failed to realize that when the worst has happened, there's nothing left to worry about. I began to see the futility of anxiety, the prison of the "what-ifs." By some grace I had been given the gift of the ability to walk completely in the moment, feeling my edges blur in some yogic fusion with the oneness of things. Eventually it wore off.

It's unfathomable really, to have survived those first two years. I did some truly tragic things. I sat on Jack's swing in the park drinking mini-bottles of vodka. I sat in his crib for hours hoping for a sign from him. I met with my rabbi demanding answers. "God cries too," he shrugged.

Thank god for Charles. "Everyone divorces over the death of a child," people said, a curse. I guess it's because the grief comes in waves and you resent your partner's suffering if you're having a reprieve. Better to cut loose and be with someone happy. But we weathered it. We held each other with the exquisite tenderness we both needed, every day.

I went to the cemetery for the first time last week, eight years after Jack died. "A life of love and joy." That's what we wrote on the stone of my turquoise-eyed precious, my little cuddle-bug, soft as a bag of feathers. Call it mother's instinct but I couldn't do it until time passed; I can deal with a skeleton.

My second son, Sam, is now nine years old. It's incredible that I had him at age 42, with IVF. It was beyond my dreams. All I wanted was a kid who'd survive. It's only recently that I can actually relax and appreciate so many unexpected qualities—his photographic memory, the maturity of his throaty laugh. Thank god for him. I'll tell him all about his brother one day.

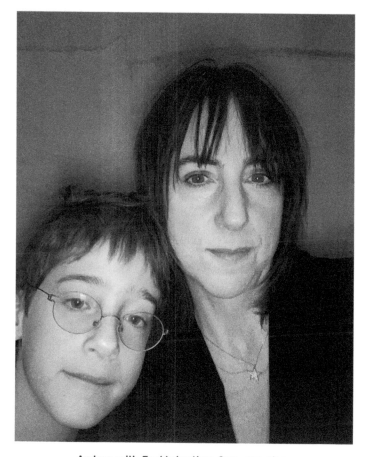

Andrea, with Jack's brother, Sam, age nine.

**Andrea Aster** is a lifelong writer, journalist and strategic communicator who currently works on behalf of a Toronto girls' school. Andrea was formerly an editor and writer at a variety of regional newspapers and magazines across Canada. She is grateful to be a happily married wife and mother. Nevertheless, she seeks opportunities for creative, solitary adventures whenever possible.

Jennifer

# How to
# Save Your
# Own Life

Finney Boylan

They placed an unlit candle in my hands as I entered the room. It was sombre in there, befitting the late autumn evening outside. Hundreds of people sat quietly in chairs. Someone was tuning a guitar.

This was at the LGBT Community Center on 13th Street in New York, at an event called the Transgender Day of Remembrance. It happens every year, people coming together to mourn trans individuals lost to murder or suicide. It's an event which always leaves me more than a little dispirited, and not only because of the senseless loss of human life the event commemorates. As a trans woman, I also wish that the one day on the calendar that recognizes transgender experience was about celebrating the successes of our our diverse community, rather than counting the lives we've lost.

On Sunday, December 28, a 17-year-old named Leelah Alcorn left her house in Kings Mills, Ohio. She made her way to Interstate 71 and waited for her moment. Then she stepped in front of a tractor-trailer. A note she left behind on Tumblr read, in part, "Please don't be sad, it's for the better. The life I would've lived isn't worth living ... because I'm transgender."

The child of conservative Christians, Leelah's parents were not supportive of Leelah's urgent pleas to begin transition and to live her life openly. "I told my mom, and she reacted extremely negatively, telling me that it was a phase, that I would never truly be a girl, that God doesn't make mistakes, that I am wrong. If you are reading this, parents, please don't ever say that to someone, especially your kid. That won't do anything but make them hate them self. That's exactly what it did to me."

The story dominated social media during the week between Christmas and New Year's, and focused not only on the suicide but on the parents' response to the child's call for help. The Alcorns took Leelah to Christian therapists, who attempted reparative conversion therapy. When that didn't work, they took away her access to social media, so that she wouldn't be able to be part of any community of like-minded souls. After the death, they took the suicide note off of the Tumblr site.

Last Wednesday, Lela's mother, Carla Alcorn, appeared on CNN to defend herself and her husband. The grieving mother denied that she is a "horrible person."

"He was an amazing musician and artist," she said, of the child she knew as Josh. "He was an amazing boy."

In the aftermath of the death, the Alcorns made no mention of Leelah's transgender identity, or even that it was a suicide. Carla Alcorn wrote on Facebook that her child "went home to heaven this morning. He was out for an early morning walk and was hit by a truck."

Some activists are calling this the "Matthew Shepard moment," the case that finally brings the plight of trans youth into the mainstream. The problem, of course, is that trans people are murdered, or take their own lives, all the time.

There was a time when I came very close to being among their number.

One day, a few years after I got out of college, I loaded all my things into the Volkswagen and started driving. I wasn't sure where I was going, but I knew I wanted to get away from the Maryland spring, with its cherry blossoms and its bursting tulips and all its bullshit. I figured I'd keep driving father and farther north until there weren't any people. I wasn't sure what I was going to do then, but I was certain something would occur to me that would end this transgender business once and for all.

I set my sights on Nova Scotia. I drove to Maine and took a ferry out of Bar Harbor. I drove onto the *S.S. Bluenose* and stood on the deck and watched America drift away behind me, which as far as I was concerned was just fine.

There was someone walking around in a rabbit costume on the ship. He'd pose with you and they'd snap your picture and an hour or so later you could purchase the photo of yourself with the rabbit as a memento of your trip to Nova Scotia. I purchased mine. It showed a sad looking boy— *I think that's a boy*—with long hair reading a book of poetry as a moth-eaten rabbit bends over him.

In Nova Scotia I drove the car east and north for a few days. When dusk came, I'd eat in a diner, and then I'd sleep either in the car or in a small tent that I had in the back. There were scattered patches of snow up there, even in May. I kept going north until I got to Cape Breton, which is about as far away as you can get from Baltimore and still be on dry land.

In Cape Breton I hiked around the cliffs, looked at the ocean. At night

I lay in my sleeping bag by the sea as breezes shook the tent. I wrote in my journal, or read the poetry of Robert Frost, or grazed around in the Modern Library's *Great Tales of Horror and the Supernatural.* I read one up there called *Oh Whistle and I'll Come to You, My Lad.* In the car I listened to the Warlocks sing *In the Early Morning Rain* on the tape deck. I thought about this girl I knew, Grace Finney. I thought about my parents. I thought about the clear, inescapable fact that I was female in spirit and how, in order to be whole, I would have to give up on every dream I'd had, save one.

I stayed in a motel one night that was officially closed for the season, but which the operator let me stay in for half price. I opened my suitcase and put on my bra and some jeans and a blue knit top. I combed my hair out and looked in the mirror and saw a perfectly normal looking young woman. *This is so wrong?* I said to myself in the mirror. *This is the cause of all the trouble?*

I thought about settling in one of the little villages around here, just starting life over as a woman. I'd tell everyone I was Canadian.

Then I lay on my back and sobbed. Nobody would ever believe I was Canadian.

The next morning I climbed a mountain at the far northern edge of Cape Breton Island. I climbed up to the top, trying to clear my head, but it wouldn't clear. I kept going up and up, past the tree line, past the shrub line, until at last there was just moss.

There I stood, looking out at the cold ocean, a thousand miles below me, totally cut off from the world.

A fierce wind blew in from the Atlantic. I leaned into it. I saw the waves crashing against the cliff below. I stood right at the edge. My heart pounded.

I leaned over the edge of the precipice, but the gale blowing into my body kept me from falling. When the wind died down, I'd start to fall, then it would blow me back up again. I played a little game with the wind, leaning a little further over the edge each time.

Then I leaned off the edge of the cliff at a sharp angle, my arms held outward like wings, my body sustained only by the fierce wind, and I thought, *well all right. Is this what you came here to do?*

*Let's do it then.*

Then a huge blast of wind blew me backwards and I landed on the moss. It was soft. I stared straight up at the blue sky, and I felt a presence.

*Are you all right, Son?* said the voice. *You're going to be all right. You're going to be all right.*

Looking back now, I am still not sure whose voice that was. My guardian angel? The ghost of my father? I don't know. Does it really change things all that much, to give a name to the spirits that are watching out for us?

Still, from this vantage point—over 25 years later—my heart tells me that was the voice of my future self, the woman that I eventually became, a woman who, all these years later, looks more or less like the one I saw in the mirror in the motel. Looking back on the sad, desperate young man I was, I am trying to tell him something. *It will get better. It will not always hurt the way it hurts* now. The thing that right now you feel is your greatest curse will someday, against all odds, turn out to be your greatest gift.

It's hard to be gay, or lesbian. To be trans can be even harder. There have been plenty of times when I've lost hope.

But in the years since I heard that voice—*Are you all right, Son? You're going to be all right*—I've found, to my surprise, that most people have treated me with love. Some of the people I most expected to lose, when I came out as trans, turned out to be loving, and compassionate, and kind.

I can't tell you how to get here from there. You have to figure that out for yourself. But I do know that instead of going off that cliff, I walked back down the mountain that morning and instead began the long, long journey toward home.

I've told this story a number of times since I came out in 2001. In 2011, I contributed a version of it to the "It Gets Better" Anthology, a project masterminded by columnist Dan Savage and his husband Terry Miller. The book, which began its life as a series of YouTube videos, intended to give young LGBT people hope in the wake of several teen suicides that year. On the whole, it's been a force for good in the world. And yet, for many young gay people, and for trans youth in particular, things don't get better.

"People say 'it gets better' but that isn't true in my case," Alcorn wrote in her suicide note. "It gets worse. Each day I get worse."

Since Leelah's story broke, I have struggled with the question of whether it does a disservice to counsel young people, trapped in unsupportive communities, denied access to treatment, to have hope. There are times when I have thought that, as Paul Simon once wrote, "sometimes even music cannot substitute for tears."

And yet I want to tell the Leelahs of the world that hopelessness is not inevitable. I came up with a list of nine things that can help save young lives.

1.  Read. Knowledge about who you are will bring you power. Two good places to start: Janet Mock's "Redefining Realness"; and Kate Bornstein's "Hello Cruel World," a book that provides a whole cornucopia of alternatives to taking one's life.

2.  Write. Keep a journal. Tell your story. It might be fantasy that helps keep you alive until you have greater control over your own life, or it might be a diary of your days. But narrative can help you make sense out of the chaos of life.

3.  Talk. Find people you can trust, and can talk to. If someone tries to convert you, or talk you out of your own truth, find someone else. The world is full of trans men and women living full and dignified lives. Find your people.

4.  Be patient. The worst thing about this condition is not having the life you want, immediately. But if you don't play a long game, you won't survive until you reach an age when your life is your own.

5.  Make noise. Do what you can to express yourself, whether it's through music or art or just standing outside and screaming. Don't keep what you feel inside. Cast a shadow so that you know you exist in the world.

6.  If you can stand it, do your homework. School can be unbearable for gender non-conforming people. But education can also be your get-out-of-jail-free card, and give you the power to take control over your life.

7.  Know that you are not alone. There are tens of thousands of transgender people in this country and we are a rising force, taking control of the narrative of our lives. You have family.

8.  If you are a person of faith, know that not every denomination is hostile. UCC and Universalist/Unitarian churches can be particularly welcoming. Look for "open and affirming" congregations. Find your people.

9. If you are in crisis, call this number: 877-565-8860, the Transgender Crisis Hotline. Or this one: 800-273-TALK, which is the National Suicide Prevention Lifeline.

That's my list, which is surely subjective, and the result of my own particular life as a writer and a musician. But there are plenty of other ways of saving your life. The hashtag #RealLiveTransAdult on twitter leads to many more stories of people who survived.

It may be possible yet to fulfill at least one of Leelah's wishes. In her note, she wrote, "My death needs to mean something. My death needs to be counted in the number of transgender people who commit suicide this year. I want someone to look at that number and say, 'that's fucked up' and fix it. Fix society. Please."

At that Day of Remembrance ceremony in November, I sat there as the speakers talked about the precious souls we'd lost in 2014. I thought, Please, not one more. I listened to a trans person play guitar and sing, and felt my eyes shining.

And then I lit that candle.


Elements of this piece have appeared previously in *The New York Times* and elsewhere. This is the first time this piece has appeared in this form.

---

**Jennifer Finney Boylan**, author of 15 books, is the inaugural Anna Quindlen Writer in Residence at Barnard College, Columbia University. She serves as the national co-chair of the Board of Directors of GLAAD, the media advocacy group for LGBT people worldwide. She has been a contributor to the op-ed page of *The New York Times* since 2007 and in 2013 she became Contributing Opinion Writer for the page. Jenny also serves on the Board of Trustees of the Kinsey Institute for Research on Sex, Gender, and Reproduction. She is a consultant and cast member for I AM CAIT, the docu-series about Caitlyn Jenner that debuted on the E! network in July of 2015 and also served as a consultant to the Amazon series TRANSPARENT.

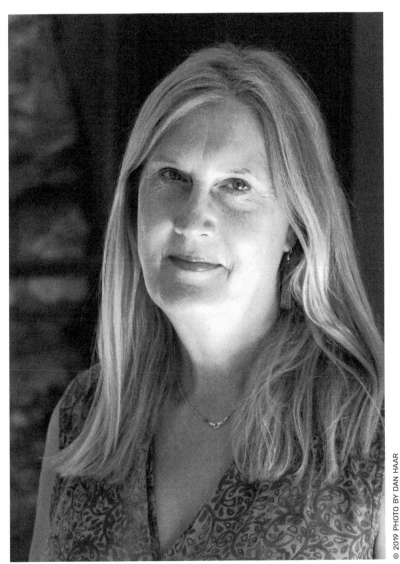

Jennifer

# Unremembered

Boyle

A high-pitched beeping sound startled me awake. I lifted my head. I was attached to a heart monitor, lying on a stretcher in a hospital emergency room. My heart pounding in my chest, my breath shallow.

*Am I losing my mind? Why can't I remember anything?*

"Ms. Boyle has been here several times in the past few weeks. She's a psychiatric patient and a frequent flyer," said a nurse.

Tears streamed down my face as I watched her scowling at the nearby nurse's station. Patients are deemed "frequent flyers" when they visit the emergency department often, for no valid reason, wasting time and resources. I had returned to the ER multiple times over the last month because I was fainting repeatedly and losing my memory.

"Hello Ms. Boyle. What brings you here this evening?" asked the doctor as she pulled aside the blue curtain.

"I'm scared. I've fainted six times since this morning."

Before I could continue, bright specks of light appeared in my vision, a constellation of stars floating in the dark. Then, my arm and leg muscles began to contract violently. Nothingness.

I wrestled to lower the side railing of the stretcher. It was the following morning, and as I lay back defeated, Dr. B, my psychiatrist, appeared and maneuvered the railing down with ease. I sat on the edge of the bed with my head bent down. My fine brown hair fell forward and shielded my face.

"Jenny, we would like to admit you to the inpatient unit," said Dr. B.

*Just another psych case, right?* "No! I want someone to take what's happening seriously." My cheeks felt hot as anger coursed through me.

"Jenny, I promise to take this seriously."

The sincerity in his voice gave me a little peace. I agreed to be transferred to the inpatient psychiatric ward.

A nurse and I walked through the twisting hallways of the hospital to the neurophysiology department. A neurologist had ordered an electroencephalogram, an EEG.

When we arrived, we were escorted into a small room with a chair in the centre.

"I'll just have you sit here, while I prepare your scalp to attach the leads," said the technician.

"Will this hurt?" I asked.

"Not at all, honey. You can sleep if you wish."

The technician glued a rainbow of wires to my scalp—red, blue, green, and yellow. She explained that the wires measured the electrical activity of my brain so neuronal activity could be tracked. Exhausted, I fell asleep in the cushioned chair.

The EEG revealed that I was not fainting as I had thought, but that I was having seizures. A wave of relief hit me. Mental illness does not preclude physical illness.

The seizures disoriented me and interfered with my ability to store memories. I could only recall fragments of my day. Once the seizures were controlled by medication, my ability to form new memories gradually returned.

The summer passed before me like a dense fog. A clear mind brought devastation when I discovered that I could no longer access the memories of my first 38 years. They had been erased. I had extensive retrograde amnesia, a condition in which a person's pre-existing memories are lost. Lost was exactly how I felt.

One morning, a young neurology resident with perfectly combed brown hair and a virtually wrinkle-free white coat entered my hospital room.

"You requested to speak with me?" he said with a sigh.

Neurologists, in my experience, were allergic to psychiatric patients. In all fairness, I was a neuro-patient, too.

"Can you explain to me why I am having trouble remembering my life, everything?"

"The brain is a complex and mysterious thing."

"Seriously? I'll need more information than that."

"You see, there are different types of memory. If memory is classified using time, it is divided into sensory, short-term, and long-term memory. Your short-term memory is improving with the anti-seizure medication, but you still have retrograde amnesia, an impairment with your long-term memory," he said.

Heather, my nurse, joined me after the resident left. We continued to talk about the different types of memory.

Long-term memory breaks down into several different types. Episodic or autobiographical memory stores all the significant events that make up our lives. Semantic memory lets us retain the meanings of words, facts, and general knowledge. Physical skills, that we have learned, fall into procedural memory. Long-term memory's capacity seems limitless, and it can last from days to years.

My amnesia affected my episodic memory, but my semantic and procedural memories were mostly spared. I was able to remember my language skills and how to do things like tying my shoelaces, but I could not remember events and experiences such as my university graduation or my sister's wedding.

"You're lucky. If your ability to form new memories continued to be impaired, you would've likely been institutionalized," said Heather.

I shivered at the thought.

Over the course of the summer, I was reintroduced to my family and friends, but I did not remember first encounters or any of the past we shared. My brother remained amorphous. He did not visit because of his strong aversion to anything medical.

"What are you doing with those index cards?" asked my sister, Holly.

"I'm keeping notes on everyone who comes to visit me. I don't want to forget them again. I need to rebuild my memory."

"What's on my card?"

Reluctantly, I replied, "Your card reads: younger sister by 4.5 years, thick brown shoulder length hair, striking green eyes—recessive gene."

I wrote the names, physical descriptions, and our connection for everyone who visited. I also tried to absorb all the information they told me about myself. My parents were divorced, my sister was married, and I was single. I thought it was fortunate that I was not married with children. The impact of my memory loss was difficult for my parents, siblings and friends, but I could not imagine explaining to children or a husband that I no longer knew them.

I met people whom I had known for 20 years and I needed help to identify them. I discovered my sister was a phenomenal resource for my personal and family lives. Maria and Angeline, my best friends, were a treasure trove of information, too. I inundated them with questions to recapture my life.

When my father came to see me in early July, he sat askew on the plastic hospital chair and twisted a gold watchband that was too big for his wrist.

"Have there been any breakthroughs today?"

"No, Dadine. Nothing. I only know that I have some sort of seizure disorder."

*Why did I call him Dadine?*

I positioned myself cross-legged on the bed.

"How are they going to fix it?"

"Medication. I guess."

"Have any memories returned? Are we going to get Old Jenny back soon?" He leaned forward as he asked the question.

"Again, Dadine, I don't know."

I looked down at my hands. I knew the man in front of me was my father, but I could not remember our history. He was the father who had raised me; I was no longer the daughter he had raised. Confusion and sadness overwhelmed me. My father's next question brought me back to the room.

"When can you return to work?" He shifted in the chair, looking like he wanted to flee.

"No idea." He wanted a breakthrough, but I had none to offer. I felt as if I had let him down, and tears threatened to take over again.

The medical team ordered an MRI. I was positioned on a narrow table with my head immobilized by a helmet. The large tunnel-like machine whirred to life taking pictures of my brain. I could hear loud clicks and bangs, even with earplugs in place. My shoulders were squished against the sides of the chamber. I had to close my eyes and count, to keep claustrophobia at bay. I needed results from the brain imaging to answer my father.

The next day, Dr. B entered my room and leaned against the far wall. Two wide-eyed medical students followed in tow.

"Hi Jenny. How are you?" he asked, looking directly at me.

"Okay," I said, my standard response to every question asked by staff.

Dr. B's calm voice delivered the news.

"Jenny, your MRI scan has shown white matter abnormalities in both of your temporal lobes. These are often referred to as brain lesions."

Silence. This revelation meant nothing to me. I understood the words and envisioned the brain as a soft, wrinkly, grey organ divided into sections called lobes. "Lesions" sounded sharp, embodying its meaning of "wound, cut or injury." I had no frame of reference. The trio looked at me expectantly.

"So now what happens?" I shrugged as if this was an everyday occurrence.

Both students, who seemed puzzled by my reaction, looked inquiringly at Dr. B.

"We have to conduct a few more tests to determine the cause of these lesions. Do you have any questions?"

"Did I do something wrong to make this happen?"

"No, you didn't. Neurons in the brain have a myelin sheath, a protective coating that, when removed, damages the neuron's ability to send signals to other neurons. Several things could've caused the brain lesions. We'll work on finding out what happened."

"Can I go home now?" I did not even know where my home was.

"Not quite yet." Dr. B smiled and left the room with his students.

I later learned that demyelinating diseases that destroy the protective coating of neurons could be caused by genetics, viruses, autoimmune reactions, medication, treatment side-effects or unknown factors. In the end, no one knew why the lesions formed in my brain. My final diagnosis was "profound retrograde amnesia" and a "seizure disorder of unknown etiology."

Weeks later my hospital bed was needed, and I was deemed well enough to be discharged. I had my bag packed before they could even finish telling me the news. I sat by the doors of the locked psych ward waiting for the buzzer to signal my freedom.

I was happy to be free of "Club Med," as my new friends called the hospital, but felt apprehensive as I sat in the back of a taxi headed home. Club Med had become more familiar than my own place. I did not remember living in my apartment, which was on the 29th floor of a downtown high rise. I found it somewhat familiar when I walked in, because I had

had accompanied day passes with my mother over the last month. A small open-concept kitchen overlooked a combination living/dining room. A door on the left led to my bedroom.

I dropped my backpack on the couch and looked out the balcony doors to see the CN Tower and the blue water of Lake Ontario in the distance. There were no clouds in the sky—just a solid blue canvas.

It was time to get to know the woman I used to be, the one who had lived here. I noticed my preference for blue accents and wood furniture. On my desk—a prominent feature of the living room—was a laptop and an organized array of blue and green files.

Photographs captured the life of Old Jenny. My family had brought photos to the hospital, which we would go through to identify the people, places, and times they represented. I pored over the images in the apartment for any spark of recognition. None came.

*Who was "Old Jenny"? Who was I, now that she was gone?*

There is no distinct date that separated Old Jenny from New Jenny. I used my discharge date in September 2008 as my "new beginning."

As a teenager beginning undergraduate studies at McMaster University, I started to experience joint pain and fatigue. Initially, my family doctor dismissed my symptoms as "growing pains," but the pain impacted my ability to study and work, and, at 20, I was diagnosed with inflammatory arthritis. My family recounted this to me to explain why my joints were painful.

Holly indicated that as a result of my diagnosis, I had chosen to attend graduate school at the University of Toronto.

"What discipline was my doctorate in?" I asked. The answer depended on the various sources of information: Cellular and Molecular Pathobiology, Cartilage Tissue Engineering, or Pathology and Laboratory Medicine.

"You were motivated by your arthritis to 'grow cells in a dish'," said my mom. This was the most honest answer of all. It crystallized my understanding that the recollections of others would be slanted by their own knowledge and memories.

In my apartment, I discovered my thesis on the shelf above my desk. I traced the silver lettering on the hard-blue cover with my fingers but could not bear to open it.

My arthritis had made it increasingly difficult to work in a laboratory because of the hand strength and movements required. Old Jenny left the lab to work in health outcomes and evaluation research. This involved switching from cell biology in a laboratory to an office job evaluating a national arthritis education program. I had worked in arthritis and disability research for seven years.

*How can anyone make up for a lifetime of lost memories?*

The questions swirling in my head made me feel scared and nauseated. I called my mom and sister, and they reassured me that we would get through this together. I curled up on the couch, fell asleep, and awoke several hours later, disoriented.

*What do I do now? How can I survive as New Jenny without a past to guide me?*

Months later, I started to experience fragments or impressions of memory. Some constructs may have been confabulations from stories retold of my past. However, there are also impressions of events, people and places that seem independent from outside influence. Sometimes, I felt apprehension, fear, love, awe, loneliness, confusion or sadness, but the details of the events were always just out of reach.

My fragile new identity was based on impressions and stories told by others. Rebuilding my life seemed daunting, almost impossible. I continued to live with the uncertainty as to whether I would lose my memory again, given that the cause remained unknown and my past unremembered.

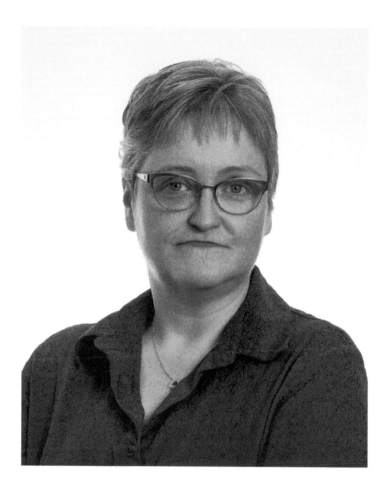

**Jennifer Boyle** is a patient advocate and volunteer for numerous arthritis-related research and educational programs. She has been involved in the Patient Partner in Arthritis program since 2010. Jennifer received the 2016 Ontario Medal for Good Citizenship and the 2018 Arthritis Health Professions Association Extraordinary Service Award for her volunteer work. Jennifer is Co-Chair of the Centre for Inter-professional Education Patient Advisory Committee at the University of Toronto. She lives in Toronto with her cat.

Steve

# Invisible
# Tracks

Brearton

On my desk is a picture of my dad and me snapped in 1969 at the botanical gardens in Thunder Bay. I'm three years old, sitting on his lap. Today, my father stares from the frame in a comforting way. The glasses he's wearing in the picture sit on my desk.

There's a second photo of my parents, with my mom, petite in a flared '50s dress, perched behind my dad. She looks so happy and holds on to him like they should never leave that time or that place. As if when they do, nothing better can happen. Their path from that moment in England led to a life in Canada with three boys and their sudden deaths outside Ottawa in 1990.

I'm 53 now and a handful of photos and my father's glasses are among the few items I have left from their lives. There's another image of my mom holding me as a bundled baby. It could be one of my brothers, but I've decided it must be my mom and me. These are the tricks we play with the dead.

My parents' death is now familiar and mostly comfortable, but there was a time it was painfully immediate. I was attending university in Toronto when my mother and father travelled by car from Ottawa to Toronto for my nephew's christening.

I was living in a shared apartment on College Street and that Saturday morning in March I walked unaware to my brother Andrew's house in Parkdale. When I arrived, I was greeted at the door by his sister-in-law. She looked panicked and when she called for my brother I knew something was very wrong. The police officer that informed Andrew of our parents' death had just left.

A drunk driver plowed into their car. He walked away from the crash. They didn't.

Two months to graduation and my mom and dad were dead. Lost to me.

When a loved one dies, those affected struggle to make sense of what happened and why, but friends and acquaintances of survivors often look for a narrative to assign death an intelligible character: paralyzed, grieving widow or bewildered orphan. It's practically a requirement of a society that emphasizes youth, rather than age, and life rather than death.

In my case, I was branded the young man robbed of the love and good guidance of my parents. Even today, people respond or reflect on my parents' death by stating "you were so young." The words unsaid, that I was abandoned or left rudderless in a difficult world. Except, I really wasn't.

I had lived away from home since age 17 and in the months immediately following my parents' death, I graduated from university and started a full-time job as a magazine editor. I was hardly abandoned. My parents had actually spent those 25 years preparing me to be independent. (Isn't that the real goal of parenting?) And during those years away from home we developed a kind of friendship unburdened by the tension and resentment that often defined my latter years at home.

And young? Before turning 25, Joan of Arc had helped oust the occupying English armies from France and been martyred, Bill Gates had cofounded Microsoft and Orson Welles had co-written, directed, and starred in Citizen Kane.

Which doesn't mean my parents' death didn't impact me. While we tend to associate crying, sadness, hopelessness and depression with grieving, men typically mourn differently. Males are more likely to experience anger, irritability, withdrawal, obsessing of the dead and too much drinking or drug taking.

I checked almost all of those boxes over the next several years. Many at the same time, but for me, I never felt a particular need to analyze death. "Death, like so many great movies," writes Dave Eggers in *A Heartbreaking Work of Staggering Genius*, "is sad."

When my brothers and I packed up my parents' home in the weeks after they perished, I was struck by how few meaningful items they left behind. I wouldn't have predicted that the single largest beneficiary of all they'd accumulated would be the local thrift shop. Their death turned into a giant jumble sale.

There were some photos, keepsakes and a few documents we kept that shed new light on their lives, like the certificate proclaiming my mom the winner of a national speed-typing contest. We took the totality of their existence and divided it into three.

My real inheritance was the time I spent with them: all those visits with my dad to the National Gallery of Canada in Ottawa or lingering with my mom in the marketplace of the Scottish town where she grew up, looking at all the fellow red heads and thinking "this is where I belong."

It's as if a life unravels and loses its form like a ball of spent wool, but the threads continue to travel beyond death through other's lives. Indigenous Australians believe in dreaming tracks or "Songlines," ancient and invisible paths that flow across land and sky and help the living navigate vast distance within the country's interior.

In Bruce Chatwin's 1987 book *The Songlines*, he writes of Aboriginal "creator beings" "who wandered over the continent in the Dreamtime, singing out the name of everything that crossed their path—birds, animals, plants, rocks, waterholes—and so singing the world into existence." Aboriginals believe the songs must continue to be sung to keep the land "alive." (My mom gave me Chatwin's *The Songlines* a few years before she died.)

I don't believe in life after death, but I do believe in those invisible tracks we lay down and a human imperative to sing the songs of those that preceded us.

So, what did the songbook my parents left me really sound like? I grew up in a house where respect, thoughtfulness, manners, responsibility and hard work were highly valued. Not surprising for parents who grew up in working-class England and Scotland during the Depression and Second World War.

What wasn't particularly admired were impromptu shows of affection or undue sharing of emotions. The latter, in particular, was frowned upon. Both were seen as signs of weakness and impediments to getting things done in life. I'm pretty sure I never saw my father cry. Keep calm and carry on were unspoken bywords in my house.

We were a white, Anglo family, in a predominantly white, Anglo society but at home we were immigrants. In the '70s, I read British publications like *Look and Learn* and soccer publications like *Shoot*, while my pals read *Owl* or *National Geographic*. When they got Lego at Christmas, I got Meccano and if their parents had weed in their freezer, we had Brussels sprouts. They ate Chef Boyardee and we ate tinned curries from Marks & Spencer.

My mom packed scones in our lunches, we ate kippers for breakfast, holidayed "back home" in the UK and my parents harboured striving new-immigrant hopes regarding integration and success for their children.

Keeping emotion in check wasn't about stifling feelings—my parents weren't cold people—it was about preparing us for life's challenges and removing what my parents saw as a barrier to success. As a child or teen-ager, I knew there was no point complaining about a teacher or a coach and expecting sympathy or some sort of action.

The message was always "stop complaining and get on with it." We were much loved and supported but rarely indulged. Working harder or better or smarter was the expected response. That also became my stock emotional response.

When my parents died, I simply didn't have the skills to process death or the language to express what I was experiencing. In fact, I had no idea what I was experiencing. I placed death in a basket together with a fight with a girlfriend or being criticized at work.

I was often overwhelmed emotionally and my response was to shut down or ignore complex demands. And it always seemed easier to listen to music and drink rather than resolve a looming problem in a relationship. Girlfriends were shut out and long-time friends ignored.

Besides, the '90s wasn't a period when people—especially people in their mid-twenties—sought advice or counseling for emotional problems. Counseling was synonymous with collapsing marriages and last-ditch efforts to convince children that every effort had been made to save the family nest. There was a stench of failure around "going to talk to someone."

Friends were supportive, but I don't believe anyone really wanted to dwell on my parents' death any more than I did. Death was largely about the small details rather than the underlying questions and conditions. "Car accident?" "Yup." "Geez." "Yup." Long pause. "God it's hot out, should we hit the patio at the Black Bull and drink some beer?"

This is the point in the story where the reader can expect to be uplifted or devastated by the resolution. Except you won't be. There's no resolution. I don't know any more about death than I did 25 years ago.

I can, however tell you a few facts: I met someone and stopped running away, got married and had three boys—just like my parents. And that's made me reflect a little on how my children will process death and what

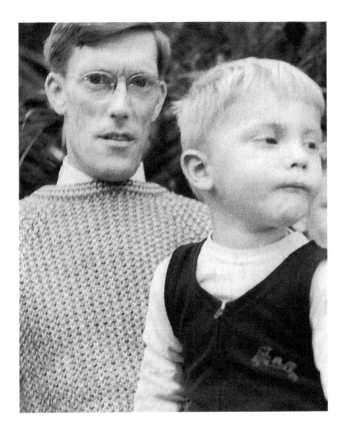

tools I will leave them to deal with the loss of their own parents. So, I've tried to be more emotionally responsive and more outwardly loving than my parents. I share more things with them, hold them and tell my three boys I love them everyday. I hope it helps them when I die.

As for death, it still makes me sad and my initial response is more acute as I get older. I'm weepier and more reflective. More sentimental. Or as my dad might have said, soft.

We like easy calculations for life, but loss doesn't equal the past sum of shared emotions or experiences, like a warehouse of melancholia we visit to remember. Nor is it the future aggregate of events never to be, a tally of sadness that grows as we carry on.

Loss is rather acceptance that we continue our relationships with the dead in a way that mirrors our contact with them when they were living. The opportunity to alter that connection in a fundamental way is gone. We invariably look backwards to death and it leaves us only with those things we started with.

I've never had *any* tidy narrative about my parents' death. And I don't always carry their passing with me. Rather, I mark their invisible tracks and I sing the songs that let me conjure my parents. I try on my dad's glasses or travel to those places my mom once stood. Then they are with me.

---

**Steve Brearton** is a magazine writer and researcher living in Toronto with his wife and three boys. Feature writer, columnist and general packager of information, he has been nominated for more than a dozen National Magazine Awards, winning Gold awards in 2003, 2007, and 2015. His work has also won the White Medal for Writing from the U.S. City and Regional Magazine Competition. Steve wore a tie to every family occasion up to age 11 and never wore a tie thereafter.

Aimee—Mishi

# We Eat
# Ice Cream for
# Breakfast

Bruner—Methven

24 June 2011.

That is "the date" for us. A month and day that had passed unnoticed in our lives for decades. A combination of numbers, unmemorable and insignificant until "that" happened. Now the date 24 June forever sends chills up my spine. It makes my stomach churn and my eyes prick with unshed tears. *That* 24 June is forever seared in my memory. Every minute of it.

I remember how we woke up at 5:15 am. The normal time, given that our two-year-old daughter Stella insisted on getting out of bed to bound into her day with the energy and destruction of the Tasmanian Devil. I remember the three of us ate cereal for breakfast, then got dressed. Aimee (my partner) and I put on our work clothes and Stella dressed herself—as always—in striped pants and a bright green T-shirt with ugly purple and pink Styrofoam sandals accessorized with orange socks.

We drove to SickKids hospital in Toronto because we wanted to get Stella's balance issues sorted out. She had recently started limping slightly and we didn't have time to wait for the specialist. We thought we would circumvent the system by getting her checked out early in the morning, get an appointment to see the specialist, then drop her at daycare and be at work by 10:00 am.

As it turned out, neither Aimee nor I went back to work for almost two years.

Hours and hours after arriving at the hospital we were given the news that made 24 June 2011 the worst day of our lives.

The doctors told us that our precious, precocious, curly-haired daughter had an inoperable, malignant brain tumour that is so terrible they use only initials to describe it—DIPG (diffuse intrinsic pontine glioma). They marched into our room, dropped that bomb on us using complicated medical terms that we couldn't quite understand, then coldly marched back out of the room leaving Aimee and I to drown in an ocean of confusion, questions and terror.

It took a few days for us to understand what they were trying to tell us—without actually saying the words to our faces.

Stella was going to die.

The child that I had carried in my womb for nine months. That we had comforted through the night. Kissed and sang to and taught to walk and talk. This girl that vibrated nothing but energy and life since the moment she burst into the world. Our only child (though Aimee was pregnant with our second), was going to die. And soon.

But before she died, we would be forced to watch her lose her faculties one at a time as the DIPG monster began to consume her brainstem, the "computer" of our bodies. We would watch her lose the ability to walk, speak, use her arms, hold her head up, swallow, and eventually breathe.

They gave her three months to live. They wanted us to radiate her tumour to "buy time." But would it cure her? "No." Could it harm her further? "Yes."

No, we decided. We would not radiate the tumour that would kill her regardless.

We would take her home. We would not waste any time at the hospital putting her through medication trials and operations. *"No!"* She would live at home with us. She would live until she died.

24 June 2011. That date was the beginning of the end for Stella and our life together.

But, it was also the beginning of our beginning.

When someone gives you news like that, it is impossible to continue to live the life you are currently living. You can no longer be upset when the line at Tim Hortons isn't moving fast enough. You can't pretend to be interested in your friend's complaint about their child not getting into the swim class of their choice. You no longer have the luxury of parenting your child for the future. Your future has been taken away. You turn inwards because you cannot exist in a world that doesn't understand what it means to live one day at a time.

And as horrible as it is to live while you are dying, there is a gift in it as well. For Aimee and I and our friends and family, we had the opportunity to do what very few people ever do: to live only in the moment. To not worry about what tomorrow may bring, because it is too overwhelming. You cut your life into smaller and smaller pieces.

Thinking months in advance is too difficult, so you talk about weeks.

Then that becomes too long-term, so you come down to days. Sometimes hours. Then minutes. Seconds.

There is a certain freedom in living a life that you know is limited. Aimee and I no longer had to worry about the "shoulds" of parenting. Stella was allowed to do whatever she wanted, whenever she wanted.

Stella ate ice cream for breakfast every morning.

And each time something was taken away from her, Stella took it right back. When she lost the ability to speak, she learned to stick out her tongue for "yes" or "no."

When she lost the ability to hold things in her hand, she grabbed a paint-brush between her teeth and created swirls of colour and life on the paper with her mouth. When she lost her ability to use her legs, she danced with her eyes.

She was never angry. Never bitter. Never discouraged.

Most importantly, she never lost herself. That mischievous, energetic girl became trapped in a body that was failing her. But she still found ways to be herself. When her baby brother was born, she delighted in "burping" him, which to her was whacking him on the back as hard as she could and laughing as he spit up on himself. She giggled when people pretended to fall and get hurt. She demanded daily pedicures and manicures from her cousin and friends. The gaudier the colours, the happier she was.

Aimee and I tried our best not to let Stella see how much we were hurting. How difficult it was to straddle two worlds. The world where we knew what was happening to Stella, where we were angry and heart-broken and jealous of our friends and their "healthy" children. And the Fairy Tale world we created for Stella where chocolate and candy flowed continu-ously, puppet shows and sing-alongs happened on an hourly basis and you could go to the park, farm, or zoo every single day.

We fed birds, went for long walks, had dance parties in the living room and a birthday party for our girl every week. Our hearts broke and soared daily. We were buoyed by our communities' wish to help us. They supplied us with copious amounts of food. Supported us financially. Brought Stella presents. Offered their time and energies to us.

We were grateful and honoured and humbled. We hosted crowds of people everyday who came to see us, to see Stella. We laughed and smiled and thanked them. We were careful not to show our deep sadness, lest we appear ungrateful or rude.

And at night, when the house was quiet and Stella slept soundly between us, we caressed her cheeks and placed our heads on her chest as we wept. We cried and raged and demanded to know why us, why her?

Then we would fall asleep holding her hands, and the next morning we would wake up with big smiles for Stella, energy and a commitment to fill this day with love and laughter because it might be the last one. We would swing the house door wide open and wait for the visits, the food, the fun to begin again.

For 16 months we lived like this. This paradox between life and death. We watched and waited. We opened our hearts to all of the lessons Stella gave us in life and resilience and gratitude. Her impact grew even as her body shriveled up.

Until finally, another date.

22 October 2012.

That was "the" day. The once insignificant combination of numbers that represents the moment Stella died, as Aimee and I held her on our bed. The day we watched her breathing slow and her limbs turn blue. The day we felt the soft weight of her for the last time as we covered her with kisses and whispered promises to her about the way we would honour her and her life.

Since then, more dates have filled our lives. Birthdays, anniversaries, firsts and lasts. And though we don't necessarily remember every single one, we do live differently now. We are not able to live life with Stella, so we live our lives in honour of her. We remember that any day can become "the" day. We spend more time playing and less time cleaning.

We read more bedtime stories to Stella's brothers. We go to the park on weeknights, "just because." We don't have "special occasion" dishes anymore. We laugh more. We cry more.

We eat ice cream for breakfast.

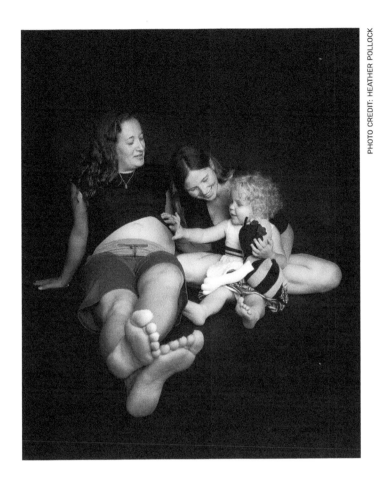

PHOTO CREDIT: HEATHER POLLOCK

Aimee and Mishi with Stella, using her puppet
Carrot to speak to her unborn baby brother, 10 weeks after
her diagnosis of DIPG (diffuse intrinsic pontine glioma).

**Aimee Bruner** is the Director of Site Expansion & Special Projects at Camp Ooch, a privately funded, volunteer-based organization that provides kids with cancer, and affected by cancer, opportunities for growth through enriching experiences. **Mishi Methven** is a Licensed Funeral Director who speaks widely about grief, bereavement and children's cancer. With Stella in their hearts, Aimee and Mishi parent Samson, Hugo, and Adele with love and ice cream.

Janet

# Grace
# Notes

Culliton

Grace was born in the small hours of a Thursday morning in late autumn, when the moon was in its waxing phase—which could trick one into thinking it was full. My obstetrician, a family friend who I had grown up calling Uncle Zol, wouldn't have said it had been an unusual pregnancy. And yet, throughout my prenatal appointments, he looked at my chart with a furrowed brow, and his right hand combed through his messy, greying hair so that it stood up on one side. It *had* been a chain of difficulties: severe morning sickness that sometimes lasted throughout the day and at times had required me to be hospitalized; the stops and starts of Grace's in-utero growth; an amniocentesis; and finally, the need for an induction when I still hadn't gone into labour two weeks after her due date.

Uncle Zol seemed especially delighted when she emerged, a healthy baby girl who had put on a little more weight in overtime, arriving at 6 lbs., 13 oz. He placed her in my arms, and I was startled to find that her eyes were open: large, dark, baby-seal eyes that locked onto mine and seemed to sear straight through to my soul. I knew in that single moment of electrical transfer that my life would be forever changed.

The next day, I asked one of the maternity nurses about the reddish purple stripes that I had discovered mapping the underside of my abdomen, now that I could see this part of my body again. The nurse was a woman from Trinidad, and she bellowed with laughter when I asked her how long it would take the welts to subside.

"Aww, honey," she said after her guffaws finally died down. "You now a mudda! Those ain't no welts! Those marks awe stretch marks, and dey might fade a tad, but dey ain't neva gunna go away!"

I burst into tears. I was emotional because of hormonal changes, and embarrassed that I hadn't known that this was what stretch marks would look like. The idea that they would not just be permanent, but so blatant—like a pronounced tattoo—had caught me off-guard. An unexpected side effect of motherhood.

I had a similar feeling of being knocked off-balance when Grace was diagnosed with autism at the age of five. This was in the years when autism wasn't so common, and doctors were more reluctant to diagnose it. It had taken two and a half years of assessments for the experts to finally make their pronouncement. The tell-tale signs of the condition—her constant bolting, her lack of accumulating vocabulary, her sleeplessness, her picky appetite, her fussiness, her limited repertoire of play-activity—all these had previously been chalked up as idiosyncrasies, behaviours that would sort themselves out in time.

Grace was, after all, intelligent—what else would explain her ability to complete 100-piece jigsaw puzzles at age two? She was highly attached to her father and me, she received and gave affection easily. And she pointed at things, something that many doctors at that time said precluded an autism diagnosis, as young children with autism aren't able to see the world from the perspective of others, and pointing assumes an understanding that others will give attention.

But the gap between Grace's development and neurotypical development had increased with each passing year. At two and a half she rode her tricycle at a fast clip for five kilometres. Around the same time, she undertook an eight-kilometre hike—running most of the way and keeping pace with her dad's fast jog through some of Ontario's roughest terrain on an old, unused county road. They scrabbled down embankments and pushed back tree branches that scratched and clawed to block the path, and then climbed up to an old road with unruly turns and a slice of elevation so steep it seemed impossible that any vehicle could navigate its ascent. By the time she got back, Grace didn't even want a rest.

In the car, or out in the stroller, she was a baby Houdini. No straps or buckles could keep her in place. She got out of her car seat and threw open the car door when we were on the highway travelling at 120 kilometres an hour. When I sat Grace down for an instant at the checkout counter to remove my wallet from my purse, her instincts for seizing the moment of distraction were razor sharp. It wasn't clear whether she had any intended destination when she made for the door with the busy main street only steps away. The impulse for her to run seemed all-consuming.

Taking her to the park, an activity that brought most mothers pleasure, was terrifying. Grace lived in constant motion, running between slides and roundabouts, climbing equipment and swings, and the road. There were always at least two or more exits to keep a watch on. My eyes followed her as though I was watching a tennis match, back and forth between Grace, the playground equipment, and the exits.

One day she swooped down the slide and used the momentum to launch herself towards an exit. I set off in pursuit, dodging parents, children, dogs and strollers in my path. I got to her just before she would have hurtled herself into the path of an oncoming car.

But the most troublesome part of her autism struck at age six. This was when Grace developed full-blown autistic rage. Her condition had suddenly become a triple threat, serving up the terror of her bolting, continual sleepless nights, and now, unimaginable levels of violence. It felt as if a giant lever had been pulled in the cosmos that opened a portal for every current of chaos and destruction to find its way into our house. There had been many previous bouts of aggression but this was on an entirely new level.

Daily life pitched between episodes of defending Grace's little sister, Ruth-Anne, from attacks, and cleaning up broken glass, porcelain, and pottery. When our available supply of breakables dwindled, Grace resourcefully found substitutes. By then, almost anything might be broken—the tea kettle, a kitchen chair, the bathroom door. The force of their impact when they came crashing down chipped the old hardwood flooring and sent splinters and wood chunks flying.

The worst violence occurred at night, when Grace stormed our bedroom. Suddenly I found myself on the floor, Grace on top of me like a wolf, ripping my hair out with her teeth, leaving my scalp bloody and mushy, and digging into my arms with her claws. And then, as though partaking in a strange cannibalistic ritual, she stuffed wads of my hair into her mouth. The struggle ended only when the wolf's energy was spent, and Grace returned to herself again, settling gently into her body and releasing her power over mine. She was dazed and docile as I led her back to her room.

One of Ruth-Anne's earliest memories was watching around the stairs to make sure Grace was not close by, so that she could descend without risk of being pushed. If Ruth-Anne was on the stairs and Grace started to come up them, Ruth-Anne turned around and locked herself in her room until Grace was up and back in her bedroom. We also taught Ruth-Anne how to secure her door each night before bed. Our sturdy house trembled when doors were smashed into or slammed shut.

I worried constantly about the effect on Ruth-Anne. How do you build a stable family life on sands as shifting as Grace's severe autism?

Sometimes, Grace cried after an incident. She crawled up on to my lap and wept tears that fell like large crystals onto her lap and mine. And we cried together, because neither of us knew what to do.

We lived this way for years. Multiple violent episodes a day, every day. Our small home looking increasingly derelict, with melon-sized holes in the drywall against which Grace had thrown her head. We sat on medical waiting lists. We told our stories over and over again. And finally, we found a combination of medications that helped give Grace better control. As the years went on, we learned some coping strategies. We amassed debt to pay for therapies, and surrounded ourselves as best we could with a network of support. But while these things reduced the number of violent episodes and helped us better deal with the ones that remained, Grace's predictably unpredictable behaviours continued to haunt us.

The trauma of Grace's earlier years has faded a little over time, just like stretch marks do, but they still are there, quickly rising to the surface on her bad days. Her tendency to have meltdowns and to be up during the night can be wearing, especially as we get older. And of course we worry about what lies ahead—how we will provide for her future, who will care for her after we are gone. The daily stress had an impact on my health. Doctors say that stress is a major risk factor for cancer, and by age 50, I had already battled cancer twice, making me worry even more about what the future might hold.

This isn't the life that any of us thought we would have, and we have struggled at times to make sense of it, holding onto the belief that there has to be something more to it than what we see on the surface. But we've also come to understand that *many* people have difficulties in their lives. It is part of what it is to be human, and we are more alike in this way than not. On the outside, other people's lives may look like the waxing moon, but it's only a trick of the eye that makes us think it is whole.

And so we have learned through Grace to be grateful for the many blessings on our own life-path. We've had some amazing helpers along the way—teachers, educational assistants, caregivers, therapists, doctors, family, neighbours and friends. And then there is Grace herself, with her sweet, tenacious spirit, the hard work she puts in every day to stay in control, the beautiful art she creates, and her smiles that have their own light source.

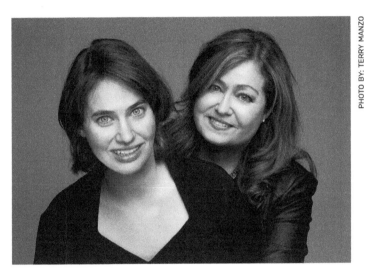

PHOTO BY: TERRY MANZO

**Grace and Janet**

Since her daughter Grace was diagnosed with autism in 1993, **Janet Culliton** has been an advocate for autism. She represented Autism Ontario on the Special Education Advisory Committee of the Huron-Perth Catholic District School Board for 15 years, received her Autism Intervener Certificate from the Geneva Centre in 2005, and has served on the Board of Directors of Autism Ontario. Janet has received volunteer service awards from the Province of Ontario and from her hometown of Stratford. She helps bear witness to the complex needs side of the autism spectrum, which remains the most vulnerable and the least helped. Despite Grace's challenges, she is an accomplished artist and has won awards for her work. Grace was the poster girl for the Geneva Centre's International Symposium in the year 2000, and received a Temple Grandin Award in 2001. Janet is a graduate of the University of Toronto's Creative Writing School.

Vicki

# All the
# Other Kids
# Died

Dunleavy

All the other kids who started chemo at the same time as me died.

It is 1975 and I'm seven years old. I'm at home. I sneak into my bed thinking I haven't been noticed. He has been drinking and yelling. Danger is around him. My mom comes into my room and says I have to go out to the living room and say goodnight to my father. As he has done so often before, he squeezes me and won't let go. He thinks it's funny but I don't like it. He holds me tight. Touching me. I try to free myself, resisting him as much as a seven-year-old can. He feels a lump on my bum. The power he has over me changes to concern. For a moment.

My days of going to school and playing in the playground end.

At the Hospital for Sick Children in Toronto everyone is keeping secrets from me. I can tell by their body language, and I hear whispering behind closed doors. I hear them say "20 percent." That is the survival rate of children with Rhabdomyosarcoma. Soft tissue cancer. I have just been diagnosed. My mom took me to the play room—cold, no fun, no smiles—at the hospital to tell me I need medicine for 18 months.

I liked the taste of medicine I've had before, so I agreed to take it, until she explained it was given through needles. That's when I said no. But I had no say in what was going to be done to me. I don't understand how this torture is going to help me.

I had two surgeries and 18 months of chemotherapy.

I'm being wheeled across the hallway to the operating room. I'm dopey and cold. The walls are white and the lights hurt my eyes. I don't understand. I don't like this.

A couple weeks ago I was in school playing with my friends. My mom says I may not have a left leg when I wake up. The surgeon will decide if he has to remove my leg. Panic, drifting toward unconsciousness. I may have said: "don't take my leg off." I remember thinking it.

My mom can't be with me when I wake from surgery. A mother of a teenage boy will be in my room when I wake up. My mother explains to me that the teenage boy was not expected to survive the night. She explains that his mom will be with me when I wake up and stay with me if her son was alive, and if he had died she would not stay with me for too long.

The boy and I are introduced. There is a look in the eyes when someone is close to death. I saw that look in his eyes. It seemed we were both thinking: "why are they introducing us?"

The boy's mother did not stay long.

I'm sad for her and alone. Scared in a cold white room.

My stay in the hospital has given me a break from the abuse at home. My mind is starting to relax. I don't need to know where my father is in the house, how to stay out of his reach.

My first roommate and I play Eye Spy. She and I laugh and giggle.

I got bored lying in a hospital bed. Since no one explained what was going on, I climbed over the side rail that was supposed to keep me in. My left leg was there, but it was not working, and I fell to the ground. My roommate presses the panic button even though I say not to, and the nurses came running in. I was afraid that I'd be in trouble, but they didn't yell at me. The nurses made sure the 18 stitches in my gluteus were holding and put me back in bed.

A couple of days later nurses came into our hospital room and drew the curtain around my bed. I knew this meant I was going to be examined. But this time, the nurses didn't acknowledge me, and instead walked over to my roommate's bed. She had been quiet the past day and had slept most of the time. I could see the feet of people underneath the curtain around my bed.

My roommate was wheeled out of our room and into a private room. That's where she died. No one said anything to me. I did not say goodbye to her. I don't remember her name. After a few more of my roommates died (... the same pattern ... curtains drawn ... hushed voices ... feet moving ...) my mom asked that I not have any more roommates.

I had stopped talking by this point.

When I returned home, my best seven-year-old girlfriend did all my talking for me, since she knew me so well. She created words and answers out of my silence.

I'm at home now and I wake with a strange feeling in my stomach. My father has left me alone lately. Maybe he will be nice to me from now on.

At home I can breathe deeply, calm my stomach.

Driving down the 401 toward Toronto my stomach starts to feel strange again. We are on the 427 southbound ramp heading toward the hospital again. My heart starts racing. Now we are almost at SickKids. My body is warm and numb. The city smells make my stomach churn. The smell in the underground parking lot makes me feel like I'm going to vomit. Faint. I'm not able to control the anxiety.

We enter the hospital and follow the yellow line on the floor to the registration desk. The cafeteria is near and the smell of the food makes me feel sick. I go to the lab for blood work and then for a chest X-ray before taking the elevator to the tenth floor, the chemo suite. I register and follow the green line on the floor to the blood lab. A scalpel blade moves toward my thumb. I tense up, hoping the nurse is able to puncture my thumb without making a slice—that's what they usually do.

Now I follow the red line on the floor to the X-ray. I have been at the hospital for two hours. There is no turning back. My heart is racing. Panic inside me, scratching. My system is pure stress. Muffled screaming inside me. The elevator ride to the tenth floor makes my stomach flip-flop. Fear squeezing inside me.

I'm tired. I just want to lay down in my bed at home. After my chemo injection I am sick to my stomach for 24 or 48 hours, depending on which of the three chemo drugs I get.

The waiting room is full. I wait two hours. I try to relax before my name is called. The game shows on television occupy my mind a bit. My name is called. I slowly walk towards the nurse. She is smiling. She takes us to the treatment room. Now we have 15 minutes to wait until the doctor comes in. My heart won't slow down. How can I stop them from doing this to me? I cry each time, trying to convince them not to give me the needles.

For the next 18 months my mom and I drive from Georgetown to Toronto for this.

In my teens and twenties I experience intrusive memories, recurrent dreams, physiological reactivity, flashbacks. Especially driving to the city, where I now live, three days a week. Elevators make me feel ill. Brightly lit rooms. Smells of the city. Anyone grabbing me in a harmless gesture, by the arm. Triggers everywhere. Even now, 42 years later. TV game shows.

Pathological effects. Physiological and psychological responses to simple things. I have avoidance symptoms (inability to recall, detachment, avoiding thoughts or feelings of the experience) which make the sensory input triggers undetectable, except to me. Intrusive vivid dreams that I remember when I wake up.

Diagnosed with PTSD by a psychologist, 2010.

The chemo injection goes into my arm, hand or foot, depending on which limb has the healthiest vein. The chemo is kept cold—I feel it trace through my veins until it warms up around my heart—I taste it as it flows up my neck into my head—my head fogs, goes numb.

I cry each time. I hope that will stop them. Sometimes the needle passes right through my vein and the plunger pushes the drug into my muscle by mistake. The muscle burns. I feel I should not have to get another needle, it's not fair, I've had enough, it was their mistake, but they give me another needle.

For 18 months I get injections. Three drugs. The schedule:

*Drug 1*—Monday, Tuesday, Wednesday, Thursday, and Friday. It does not make me vomit, but it makes me nauseous and stoned. The stress of the drive into the city, to SickKids. I miss school for the week.

*Drug 2*—Four Thursdays in a row. This one makes me sick for 24 hours and stoned. I miss two or three days of school.

*Drug 3*—Every other Thursday during the month. This one makes me sick for 48 hours. It's the hardest to recover from. I miss three to four days of school.

They take bone marrow from my spine without an anesthetic. I scream in pain. A six-inch needle is inserted up my spine from my tail bone. There are four adults holding me down, restricting my movement. I'm told if I move

I can be paralyzed. I channel the pain through my screams and hold still.

They come in waves, without warning. Memories I try to suppress.

In 2000 I had a dream that I was a child in the hospital. A black-and-white movie. I watched myself. The dream was real. I woke up. While I was dreaming I started worrying about my daughters. Before I could fully wake up, I thought I must be dreaming because if I was eight years old and in SickKids I wouldn't have kids of my own. My consciousness grasping for logic to stop the panic.

In 1975 there were no support programs for kids with cancer. It wasn't spoken about. I didn't have an outlet to process fears. At age eight I realized it was up to me to survive. I learned I would be okay by myself. As an adult it leaves you feeling comfortable when you are alone. But I don't want to be alone.

It is 2016. I've been told a dear friend is going to die in a week. I start to feel I'm spinning out of control. Inside. I can feel *it* but I'm not clear on what *it* is.

I try to process the news of my friend dying but I feel the disorder coming. My friend is not going to be with me in a week. A new trigger.

When I was eight, my roommates died. For a week I feel worse each day, wanting to be alone, isolating myself from close friends. They are aware that they should keep in touch with me, and they do, but I turn down invitations to spend time with them.

I start to dissociate my mind from my body, like I did during my cancer treatment. I go through the days trying not to feel. The *it* became clear in a dream. A black-and-white movie that I'm watching and acting in. I'm now familiar with these dreams.

I am a child in the hospital. Doctors are giving me a needle, saying I'm going to die. I didn't want to die. I say I want to play with my friends.

The doctors told my "parent"—my adult self in the dream—that I would owe them three million dollars for the drugs if I didn't let them give me the needle.

I wake up before the needle.

I have been living with this heightened fear of dying for the past 42 years. I exercise regularly to stay strong—to keep off the fear of dying.

If I feel physically weak, my brain thinks I'm sick and dying. Medical marijuana reminds me to eat and lowers my anxiety. My brain is conditioned to override hunger signals. Chemo treatment made me sick to my stomach. I wouldn't eat even if I was hungry, since eating made me vomit.

It's been like going through life in a daze. I have made some wrong decisions.

When I was a child I was afraid I was going to die soon, and I didn't want to die. I discovered at the age of age eight that the best way to cope was to repeat the mantra, "I'm not going to die." This won't work when I am older and closer to death.

My father started to abuse me again after I'd finished chemotherapy and had recovered.

A friend's mother was a social worker—she took me from my parents' house when I was 15. I fought to protect myself from my father, but I was only a kid.

That is a different story.

———

**Vicki Dunleavy** is the mother of two daughters, and has one granddaughter. She lived in Toronto but had to move back to Creemore full-time in September 2017 because of her PTSD. She is a participant in the Long-Term Follow-Up Study through St. Jude Children's Research Hospital, which tracks adult survivors of childhood cancer diagnosed between 1970 and 1999. Vicki volunteered in oncology at the Royal Victoria Hospital in Barrie but had to stop because her PTSD symptoms worsened. In 2010 she rode her bike across Canada as part of the Sears National Kids Cancer Ride. She is the personal assistant to Morden Yolles. She plays piano and hockey, and enjoys cycling, hiking and weight training. She would like to become a trainer of dogs for PTSD patients, and in 2018 she trained a dog for herself, a German Shepherd named Willow.

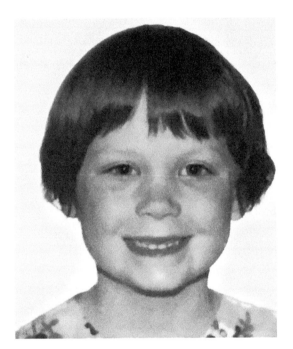

Vicki Dunleavy, just before she was diagnosed.

Janelle

# Walking
# as I Wake

A. Girard

Cement walls narrow into a hallway. The only light comes from street lamps gleaming through double-glass doors. Each exit is perfectly spread out, every 20 feet, with its own numbered panel hanging overhead. Toronto's Union Station bus terminal is empty of everything but the maturing scents of the month of May.

The balls of my feet ache. I look down. I see that I am walking barefoot. My right hand clings to the shirt that I had put on after the gym. My legs are bare. Where are my skinny jeans? I am soaking wet. I try one of the platform doors, but it's locked. My pulse races. Eyes heavy, sight blurry, awareness cloudy. As though just awaking from sleep but with no recollection of ever having gone to bed. I stumble over my feet. My arms fly out to my sides in an attempt to steady my body, but the walls are too far for my reach. My palms pound the cold concrete floor. Breath short. The air is beginning to thicken with humidity. It is becoming increasingly harder to breath.

"Excuse me Miss, are you alright? Are you hurt? Let me help. We're EMS."

Emergency Medical Services come out of nowhere. How did they get in here? I can't even get out.

"No, no, I'm fine, thanks. Just need to get a cab and get home."

I hear my voice, but it's foreign. Distant. Lost.

"Miss, why don't you come with us so we can make sure you're okay."

Two paramedics approach me. One offers an outstretched hand and the other follows closely behind, carrying an orange box. I take the helping hand and allow it to lead me out of the tunnel I have been roaming for an unknown amount of time. The darkness in the sky confirms that it's night. The air is cool. My eyes acclimatize to the changes. The downtown streets are lined with locked storefronts and a few taxicabs. For a sliver of a second I marvel at the city's stillness. At the curb the ambulance awaits.

"Really, I'm okay," I say.

Tears start to gush without warning, causing the panic to swell. I feel my body being lifted onto a gurney, which has magically appeared. I don't resist the light push on my shoulders to lay me down. Something is draped over my near-naked body. I feel a strap cross over me and hear the snap of a buckle. I'm lifted up and glided along, now inside the ambulance's cavity.

I squint at the bright lights. My chariot is filled with rows of drawers and compartments of tools used to save peoples' lives. One of the paramedics takes my hand.

"Just don't turn on the sirens, okay? Please, just don't. Please. I'm not dying, I promise."

The sound of the sirens would mean there's an emergency; that I'm in danger. It would mean there's cause to panic. And with that, my mind's internal troops take me away to an oblivious state, not of sleep but of proximity.

My fingers touched the cold leather-like covering on either side of my body. As I sank deeper into the single mattress, I realized this wasn't my bed. The fog started to lift from my mind. I began to search for memory. Memory of where I was. I couldn't find the surface of my thoughts. Slowly, I brought my right leg, then my left, over the side of the bed, trying to get my bearings as I sat up. I wished I could retreat back into unconsciousness. The fingers of my left hand tapped an anxious melody: thumb, pinky, index, ring, middle—thumb, pinky, index, ring, middle—repeat.

The door to my tiny white-walled room opened. I heard chatting over charts, doctors being paged, the smell of antiseptic and the reflection of a rising sun on a dull pastel-painted wall.

A middle-aged Hispanic woman entered the room.

"Hi, I'm Detective Reyes. How are you feeling Janelle?"

*How did she know my name?*

"Do you know where you are?"

I don't answer.

"You were brought in by EMS to the Urgent Care Center here at Women's College Hospital. You're in a private room in the Sexual Assault Domestic Care Center."

The words "sexual assault" bounced against the inside of my brain like a ball inside a sphere. Bad. Very bad.

"Do you remember anything from last night?"

I dodged her question with glazed eyes, arms wrapped around my torso as tightly as possible. My skin was sore. I had no memory. No account of time. Nothing of what had happened between leaving the bar last night and being found by the paramedics. Drowning, my mind thrashed about, trying to find anything that it could latch on to.

The detective sat in one of the bucket chairs adjacent to my bed.

"The police found your jeans out in the Annex and your purse and shoes in the parking lot of the Summerhill LCBO. That's almost three kilometers apart, in opposite directions. You were found incoherent, not fully conscious of your whereabouts and half naked, roaming the bus terminal at Union Station early this morning. That's another three and a half, close to four kilometers south of those two neighborhoods. Do you remember being in any of those places?"

I stared at her blankly.

"How about we start with what you do remember," she said.

Her glance passed the conversation over to me. I shuffled in my seat and the thin-paper layering on the bed ruffled, tearing a little, and making just enough noise to own the awkward moment of silence. Detective Reyes closed her notebook and tucked away her pen.

I recounted going to the gym after work and then meeting up with my friend for dinner at Hemingway's, a pub in the upscale Yorkville district. When we were done eating, we joined two buddies of mine from high school that I had spotted at the bar for some drinks.

"What did you have to drink?" she interrupted.

"Wine."

"How many glasses?"

"Two with dinner."

"And how many with your friends at the bar?"

"Maybe another two."

"Hmmm."

*Was she keeping track of my beverage tally?*

"What made you leave the bar?" she asked.

I closed my eyes, picturing myself back at Hemingway's.

"I wasn't feeling right. I felt off, weird. It started when I caught sight of my reflection in the washroom mirror. I looked blurry. When I came back to the bar where the guys were standing, I knew I had to leave. Right away.

I couldn't see my girlfriend so I told the boys to let her know I had to go. I could feel myself drifting. But I wasn't drunk."

I opened my eyes and looked right at her.

"Sure, I buzzed, but that wasn't it," I continued. "This was different. I wasn't in my body anymore, like I was being pulled by something, away. I remember feeling the cold of the railing as I made my way down the stairs, I knew I was gripping it, but it felt more like my fingers were gliding along. I knew I was going in the right direction towards the exit because it was the only light I could see. I hit fresh air. I turned left and headed for Bay Street to get a cab."

I gripped my knees under my chin and started to sway. Nausea began to whirl in my gut. My pulse racing. Everything was spinning.

"I, I just needed to get home."

I gulped short inhales followed by crisp exhales. My hands trembled. Pieces of memories played on fast forward. Others in slow motion, over and over again. I was unable to push pause. Tears began to escape my eyes slowly at first, and then urgently.

"How about I let you rest before you go for your rape kit. We'll talk again after that."

She smiled as she rose from her chair, the only audience to my decomposition. I reached for the garbage can and vomited.

Within 24 hours, I was back at work as a French teacher for an urban private school, across the street from the bar where I was the night before. I sang songs about bubbles, explained grammar rules and made mad dashes to the photocopier while wearing an uncharacteristic amount of make-up to cover the blue-purple bruises that splotched my face.

Two weeks later, I found myself awake at 3:00 am, gulping from the bottle of wine I had stashed under my bed in the hopes of knocking myself unconscious long enough to get some imageless sleep.

Three weeks after that, I was vacationing on the beach of Cancun, Mexico, where I allotted this trip as my two weeks to get better.

Five weeks later, I was sitting on my best friend's pleather couch on a pilgrimage back to Halifax. I had gone to university there, and it had given me a confidence that I constantly fed upon to portray myself as the capable adult I had been, and now only pretended to be. I began to weep silently while everyone else slept. I was struggling to fake survival.

I wanted to be told that it wasn't my fault. That the leftover memories were going to fade soon. That the nightmares were going to disintegrate to moments of bothered sleep. To be freed from the flashbacks laced with faceless antagonists. The short, crisp staccato screeches. The thrashing.

I wanted to be told that I was still strong, and for that I should still be proud. Instead, there was judgmental silence, discreet embarrassment, and the awkward self-plea to "just get over it." I had hoped that two weeks in the sun would tan my body enough to rid me of the leftover bruises, that Halifax would bring back soothing memories and love of far-away friends.

27 May 2009. The day I was locked away where only I could feel the torture. I would never again know darkness to be so safe.

Only later would I come to understand that this wasn't my fault. I was mourning.

PTSD, chronic and reoccurring depression, ongoing anxiety, addictive tendencies, fear of the dark.

I'm still alive.

But I have neither forgotten, nor am I free. I have no small coloured ribbon to pin on my jacket to signify my ongoing battle. I have never received a standing ovation for continuing to be present and functioning as a contributing citizen of society. I have never been honoured with a medal or trophy for enduring being drugged, abducted, and sexually assaulted. They stole my clothes, took my purse, robbed me of my confidence. They beat me of my trust and my true smile. They murdered all that I had been.

But they still couldn't win.

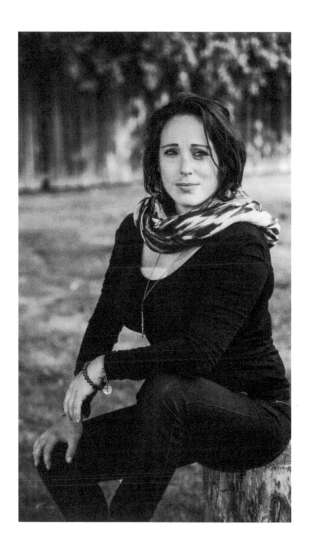

**Janelle A. Girard** received her B.A. from Dalhousie University, Nova Scotia, and her B.Ed. from OISE, University of Toronto. She has over 15 years experience teaching in both English and French from the primary through to senior grades, as well as adults and government officials, in both the private and public sector. Janelle completed her Creative Writing Certificate at the University of Toronto School of Continuing Studies in 2017. She lives in Toronto with her rescue dog, Matheson.

Lynn

# To My
# 17-Year-Old
# Self

Gluckman

The day is hot and bright and beautiful. I am lying on the beach, listening to classic rock, appreciating the lazy warmth of the Tel Aviv sun. There are probably 20 of us, Canadian students, together that day. We are relaxed, mindless from the heat. An idyllic scene: smooth sand, blue sea, happy people, idle chatter, bodies in various states of dress and undress.

And then ...

A boom—quick and deep and loud—like the sonic boom of a fighter jet moving faster than the speed of sound. But it is much, much closer. A few feet away. The sound lasts the length of a quarter note. My ears pound, deep inside. An echo that stays in the memory forever.

The vibration lifts my body off the ground. I land with a thud. I am no longer in the spot where I started. I'm in the air for a split second, but it seems like forever. Time passes in slow motion.

The sky is no longer blue. A cloud envelops the area. Is it smoke? Is it sand? Is it both? A blanket of sand surrounds us, in every direction. So much sand it distorts the scene. Pain striking against my skin.

People are screaming. Scrambling. Bodies in confusion. My instinct is to run. I run away from the chaos.

I run back to my hotel across the road. Do I take the stairs to my room or the elevator? I seem to remember taking the stairs—I did not wait for the elevator. I needed to keep running. One foot in front of the other.

I am back in my room with my friends who weren't with me on the beach. I don't have to explain what has happened: our balcony overlooks the very spot where I was lying. People running everywhere. An ambulance? Who is being taken away?

I'm shaking. I'm unclear about what just happened. I don't remember the moment I realized it was a bomb. Did others tell me? I learn later that a pipe bomb was planted beneath the sand a few feet from where we were lying. A calculated act of destruction. A terrorist attack.

I get dressed and walk out of the hotel to find a phone booth to call home. Half-way around the world, on a student tour of Israel, I need the comfort of home. I want to let my family know that I am alright. I leave the hotel and see a gaggle of reporters—CNN and others.

I find a phone booth and attempt to make a collect call. My parents are not home. The time difference means that they are likely on a golf course in Toronto. I am incredibly frustrated that I am unable to reach them. 17-year-old frustration. I try to make another collect call to my brother and his wife. They are not home. By some small miracle, the operator lets me leave a message on their answering machine even though no one has accepted the call (a merciful act of kindness on the part of a random Israeli telephone operator who likely knew what was going on, heard my North American accent, and made a judgment call).

I leave a message for them that I am okay. I don't mention any details about what has happened—I don't want to scare them. I repeat: I am okay and my friends are okay and I will call them later.

Back at the hotel, our group is called together by our tour leaders. We are told that a member of our group has been injured in the explosion. She had been taken to the hospital and is in surgery. A few hours later we are told that she has died.

Gasps. And tears. And many more tears. Tears of disbelief. I feel sick to my stomach. I am shaking, and numb.

The next few days are a blur. There are several weeks left of our trip and I have to decide. Should I stay on in a country where I no longer feel safe? Or go home? The first two weeks of the trip have been spent on a kibbutz, so I have not seen any of the country that I travelled so far to visit and to learn about. My parents do not insist that I come home early. They leave the decision up to me.

I feel a deep sense of frustration. I want to hear them tell me to come home. I want them to demand it. I realize later that it must have been incredibly difficult for them because I'm sure they wanted me home more than anything in the world. But they wanted it to be my decision and they wanted me to reach it independently. (As a parent of young children today, I don't believe I would have the emotional fortitude to react the same way.)

I am 17 years old, indecisive, not able to fully grasp the magnitude of the situation.

I did not know it at the time (and am only realizing it now, for the first time) but my contemplating to stay may have been the beginning threads of a character trait: wanting, needing to put one foot in front of the other, and continue forward in the face of adversity.

The terrorist attack on 28 July 1990 felt like the end of the world to me. I was gripped by sadness and disbelief. Why was I lucky enough to survive, while a girl my age a few feet away was not? I wallowed in self-pity. I questioned the "fairness" of life. How could this have happened to her? To me? To us all? Is it possible to have faith in a world where people could be so evil and exact such harm? Weighty existential questions to be facing a 17-year-old.

The event made me more fearful. The lens through which I viewed my life narrowed. I began to expect random and horrible events to take place in my life. If something so arbitrary and terrible could happen that day, then surely it (or something less arbitrary but equally terrible) could happen again ... and again ... and again.

But the impact did not stop me from moving forward. My family and friends helped me through. (My parents encouraged me to see a therapist, but my 17-year-old self had no desire or inclination for that.) They gave me space and time to process what had happened, but they did not allow me to wallow in my sadness or be overcome by my fears.

There were many occasions, after that day, where I would be surprised by a distinct and sharp sound that was close enough to the sound of the bomb to elicit an overwhelming reaction from me. A firecracker exploding. A balloon popping. They immediately brought on tears and trembling. Reactions were acknowledged, but never dwelt on.

Moving forward. One foot in front of the other.

Although my life would never be the same, it was quickly and very much back to "life as normal." Life does go on, which to me seemed equal parts cruel and kind.

I went to school, worked part-time, pursued my interests and passions. I went on to university and then law school. I worked hard and achieved success. I met and married my wonderful husband and gave birth to two phenomenal human beings.

And then ...

When I was in my thirties, my mother battled ovarian cancer. It is a brutal and relentlessly debilitating disease that ultimately took her life.

I underwent genetic testing and learned that I had the BRCA2 genetic mutation, which would significantly increase my risk of ovarian and breast cancer. What would that mean for my future and the future of my family?

I underwent various health screenings and exams. Many false positives and much further testing later, it wreaked havoc on my (already fragile) mental state. At the age of 41, I had preventative surgery to remove my ovaries and uterus, putting me into immediate and early menopause. At the age of 43, I had a preventative double mastectomy.

The decision to undergo these procedures was surprisingly easy for me. In fact, I would say that it wasn't a decision at all. I was armed with certain knowledge and with the tools to do something about it. That may sound clinical, but that is reality.

The operations were major and the recovery was not easy. Pain. Discomfort. Exhaustion. Fear. But they were temporary. And for the greater good.

I believe that the event on 28 July 1990 (and others after it) armed me with certain coping tools. It gave me the knowledge that I could survive difficult times and even thrive afterwards. It also allowed me to understand the power of momentum. Moving forward, taking action—whether as an unintentional coping mechanism or as a strategic approach—was necessary for me. It still is.

And then ...

Less than a year after my mother died, my beloved husband Andrew— my best friend and my rock throughout all of my trials and tribulations— was diagnosed with a rare form of recurrent brain cancer. He was 41.

I remember getting the phone call. Andrew had a seizure while working out at his health club. I was in a complete panic. An ambulance took him to the hospital, where the doctors assumed he was merely dehydrated from his workout. As a strong, healthy and vibrant man, the doctors were going to discharge him without any real investigation.

In speaking to him on the phone, I knew that something wasn't right. I was asking him questions and he had no memory of certain events. I urged the doctor to do more testing. I raced to the hospital and as I got there, the doctor delivered the test results. The scans showed that there was a large mass in Andrew's brain. I felt the blood drain from my body. Darkness enveloped me. I felt physically weak and sick to my stomach. I put my head on his shoulder. He held my hand.

Grief. Torment. Sleeplessness. Fog. Anxiety. Utter fear. Sorrow. And yet.

Now—eight years, one surgery, three rounds of chemotherapy and one round of radiation later—Andrew is faring well.

Those who know me would describe me as generally happy and positive. That is how I feel on most days. I can get through dark and difficult times. I can even do so with laughter and joy. Gratitude plays a large role in my ability to do this.

I am grateful for many things, mostly for my family and my friends. I am surrounded by caring and kind people, who have been there for me in a multitude of ways over the years. They are there to celebrate triumphs and victories—great and small—and there to help through our struggles.

I am buoyed by the humanity I have been shown on a daily basis. So many offers of help and support. Beyond the phone calls and emails and visits. There have been countless meals delivered to our doorstep. There has been assistance with childcare that has lightened our load and many other random acts of kindness. Leaving my house one day, I realized that the empty urns that stood outside our door—that I hadn't had time or energy to even think about—had been filled with the most beautiful flowers. In the weeks after Andrew's diagnosis, not having the strength or desire to think about decorating our house for Halloween, without my asking, a family friend did this for me with my children. Thoughtful and caring neighbours and friends have shoveled our driveway during winter storms. Small acts, but the impact is enormous. They are what keep me positive. And fulfilled.

I went from questioning the basic decency of humanity when I was 17 to being thankful for it at 47.

Since that horrific day, I have endured many difficult struggles. Each one has given me strength that has carried me through the next one.

To my 17-year-old self I would say: "With time and perspective and wisdom, this event will shape your life in positive ways. It will allow you to understand how strong you really are. It will open you up in ways you never thought imaginable. It will lead to your faith in the kindness of humanity. It will reveal how to put one foot in front of the other, so you can move forward with grace and humility. It will help you recognize that life's most profound challenges can allow you to truly appreciate all that is wondrous and beautiful."

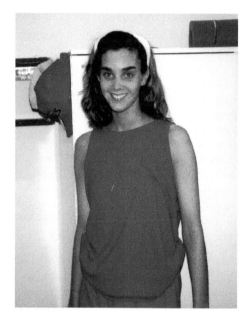

Lynn Gluckman, age 17, in Israel just days before the attack.

**Lynn Gluckman** lives in Toronto and is the mother of two remarkable young men, 12 and 16, and wife to an inspiring, rock star of a husband. Lynn practiced corporate law with a large Bay Street firm for several years, where her practice focused on mergers and acquisitions, private equity funds, and bank financing. She now works for a boutique law firm practicing exclusively in the area of non-profit and charity law. Lynn works on community fundraising events—including one run by her children in support of The Princess Margaret Cancer Centre. Recently, Lynn and her husband founded the charity www.toughsob.org that gives free, empowering toques to cancer patients. She is an amateur photographer, and a lover of music, good food and great company.

Trevor

# A Long,
# Bleak
# Christmas

Greene

I spent the winter of 2009 with metal rods drilled into the bones of my feet and into my shins, pulling my contracted feet flat, but I forget the pain. In the spring of 2008 I felt and heard my right femur snap in physiotherapy—a muffled crack of bone beneath the skin—but I forget that pain.

The severe PTSD episodes I went through in the long, bleak Christmas of 2007, however, are seared into my subconscious. At one point I tried to kill myself by stuffing my fist down my throat.

I was at one of Canada's best brain injury rehab facilities, in the tiny Alberta town of Ponoka. Somebody had given me a goofy fur hat with tie-down ear flaps that year. When the black dog howled, I'd pull the hat tightly around my head and moan softly. I had hallucinations that I was standing in a corner by our bookshelf hugging myself tightly. Even now, writing these words over a decade later, I get a sick feeling in my gut.

Ever since I had learned to read as a little boy, I had played a game of dissecting long words into short ones. I would break down "reincarnation" into "rein" and "carnation." "Mumbled" into "mum" and "bled." My mind would casually indulge my OCD at odd moments, but that winter of 2007 a tornado of words swirled inside my head. The game droned on and on anytime I wasn't occupied, and especially when I was trying to relax. Physiotherapy sessions would usually leave me winded, exhausted, but I also struggled to catch my breath at other times throughout the day as my anxiety sucked the air out of my lungs. Even my breath was not my own.

In early October, my wife Debbie and my two-year-old daughter, Grace, moved into a house near the rehab centre. I immediately asked to see pictures of the house—a big mistake. As I lay awake, cold and lonely in my bed, I thought of them warm and snuggly in a cosy home. To me it might as well have been at the North Pole. Debbie and Grace finally had a home, but there was no way to get me there. And even if I reached the house, there was no way to get me up the steps to the front door.

My good friend, Clare, and Debbie's mum, Judy, visited for my birthday in mid-November. Judy gave me a Christie Blatchford book about stories of Afghanistan, the story of my 2006 attack included.

An axe splitting my head in two—the coma—learning to move one finger at a time—speaking one word at a time.

Now that I was actually reading about the attack first-hand, my reaction was visceral and panicked. As the weeks passed, the anxiety got worse. I would become extremely agitated if I saw a uniform on TV or in person.

By December, I couldn't keep anything down. I was throwing up so regularly that Debbie had to stand by with a bucket during physiotherapy sessions, waiting for the inevitable. I became irrational and demanding. I lost control over my body as it stiffened in response to my mind's ever-increasing agitation. I shunned newspapers and TV to avoid any mention or image of Afghanistan. A glimpse would trigger a surge of terror, causing my body to go as stiff and straight as a board. A sharp pain would shoot through my abdomen as my chair's seatbelt dug in from the violent stretch.

Starved of images and current events, my mind wandered into my storehouse of memories—the most vivid of which were from Afghanistan. I would once more be hyper vigilant and claustrophobic in the dusty belly of the LAV, trying to peer through the thick armour for signs of an IED.

Psychological trauma from combat has always carried a tinge of cowardice. In World War I it was known as shell shock, and the injured were sent to field hospitals that specialized more in injuries to the flesh than to the mind. In World War II it was known as battle fatigue, and the injured were immediately pulled from combat and sent home in disgrace.

The condition is now known as post-traumatic stress disorder, PTSD. The specific military name is operational stress injury, OSI. It is as insidious and damaging as a wound to the body. Many of our soldiers return from Afghanistan more or less physically whole, but emotionally, mentally, psychologically, and spiritually shattered. Many commit suicide. My OSI was compounded by my own reality: I couldn't do anything for myself, couldn't go for a run to blow off steam, and I didn't know if I'd be in the wheelchair for the rest of my life.

The deep anxiety started with a feeling of helplessness, as if I was hearing Grace scream from the inside of a burning house and there was nothing I could do about it. Then came a feeling of rats gnawing at my stomach, their heads shaking violently as they greedily ripped into my flesh. When they started ripping into my heart, it felt as if I would never breathe again. I begged Debbie and the staff to get me to the house so I could crawl up the porch steps to the front door. The eventual gift of a wheelchair van saved my sanity. I hoped that spending five days at home with Debbie and Grace over the Christmas holidays would ease the pain.

One of the nurses at the centre had offered to buy a Christmas present for Debbie for me. I selected a diamond ring. With the help of my recreational therapist, I made a teapot in the ceramics room, then arranged for her to put the ring in it and place it under our tree. I had originally proposed to Debbie on my knees in 2005 at her grandmother's house, and I'd promised her a ring when I could get one. The thought of giving Debbie the ring, and of spending my first Christmas of memory with Grace, kept the rats at bay temporarily.

I was overjoyed when Debbie and Grace picked me up to go home four days before Christmas. I looked forward to living together in the same house, to being a more or less permanent fixture in Grace's life. I loved the house the minute Debbie pushed me through the front door. There were Christmas knick-knacks, and an undecorated tree stood in a corner of the living room. I looked forward to christening my new recliner and being close to my family over the holidays. That night, we had dinner together, and Debbie and Grace decorated the tree under my ornament-placement guidance.

On Christmas morning, Grace crawled up on my bed and we opened our stockings. Because I took too much time opening my small wrapped presents, she joyfully opened them for me. Later, as we unwrapped the gifts under the tree, I felt Grace's joyful squeals seep into my bones. I willed Debbie to tear her gifts open quickly so she could get to the one that would finish off a proposal I had started two years ago and a million miles away. As she carefully unwrapped the box and pulled out the teapot, I was overwhelmed by thoughts of what she had endured to stay by my side. Many times I had worried she would leave me. I couldn't think of a greater test of compassion and love than what she had been through. I had practised over and over the words I would use to ask this wonderful woman the most important question of our lives. I ended up winging it.

"Bee, when I could kneel, I fell to my knees and begged you to marry me. I said I would get you a ring when I had the money. Now that I have the money but can't kneel, I want you to picture me on my knees and promise you will marry me." As she wrapped her arms around me, I whispered in her ear, "I promise you I will walk down the aisle one day with you."

Throughout my five blissful days there, I alternated between swimming with joy and drowning in despair. There was the goofy, fuzzy black hat with fold-down flaps that cover ears and face. Many times I pulled the hat tight over my head and sought serenity in the darkness.

Up to Christmas, I had dealt with my painful anxiety by shutting down and shutting out the world.

In January, I cracked. The hunger of the rats, and my breathlessness, were more than I could bear. Desperate, I tried to end my life by ramming my fist down my throat, but I had neither the range nor the strength to reach far enough. The only outlet for my broken body and soul was my voice. My mind took over, and foul words spewed from my lips. As I cursed and raged at the top of my lungs, a calm, rational voice spoke softly in my head: "This is what it's like to go insane."

I howled. I was cursed and was going to hell. I wanted to go back to Afghanistan so my attacker could finish the job—I knew he was dead but that didn't stop the rage or the raging. "This is what it's like to go insane." I was shocked that such violence could erupt out of me. I had never sworn at Debbie, ever. Once, I even swore at my precious Grace. Fortunately, my voice wasn't loud enough for her to understand, and Debbie deflected it expertly, saying, "Daddy said to have a good nap."

That was over 10 years ago. I have had regular panic attacks since and wake every day with a low-level murmur of anxiety in my gut that gets worse if I get stressed. I can't have my back to a door and I hate fireworks, especially a hand-held firework that sounds like a rocket-propelled grenade. Twice a month, I attend a peer OSI group and have regular sessions with a psychologist.

My hair hides the dents in my head, and the deep scars on my feet are fading.

I can only hope that time will quiet the howls of the black dog.

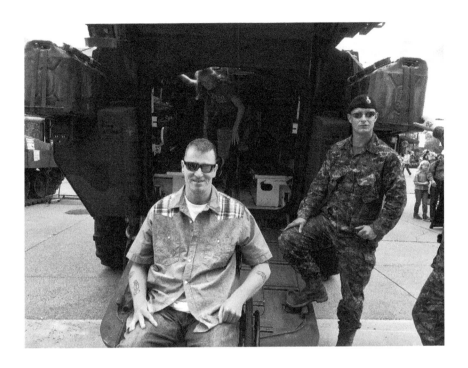

**Trevor Greene** is a journalist and the best-selling author of six books. In 1995 he joined the Canadian military and in early 2006 he was a member of the first Canadian battle group to deploy to Kandahar. On 4 March 2006, as he was meeting with local elders at the tiny riverside village of Shinkay near Kandahar City, he had put aside his weapon and took off his helmet as a sign of trust and respect. A Taliban insurgent came up behind him and drove an axe into his head. He has undergone extensive surgeries and spent a year in hospital and over a year in a specialized brain injury rehabilitation hospital. In 2010, a stranger willed $100,000 dollars to Trevor, which he and his wife Debbie used to set up a foundation, The Greene Family Education Initiative, which funds the education of girls in conflict zones. He lives in Nanaimo with his wife, son and daughter.

Teva

# Still
# Here

Harrison

# Still Here

AT FIRST, I TOLD NOBODY—I WAS ALONE WITH CANCER

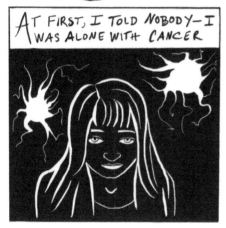

BUT SOMETHING IN ME BROKE & I NEEDED TO CONNECT—

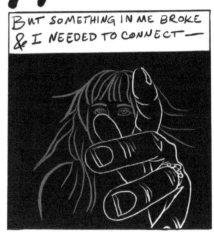

A COMMUNITY OPENED UP TO ME...

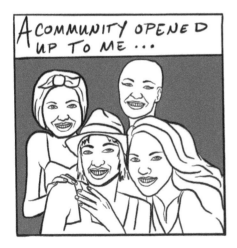

EACH WOMAN WAS MORE BEAUTIFUL THAN THE LAST

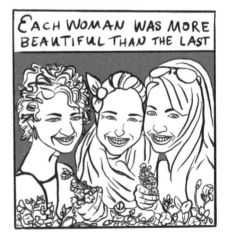

AND WE ALL SHINED OUR LIGHTS EXTRA BRIGHT, FACED WITH METASTATIC CANCER

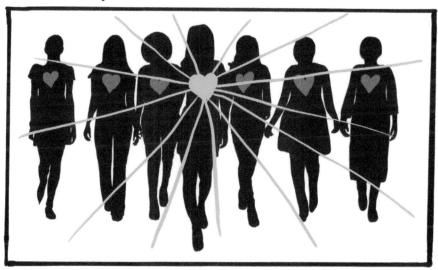

MY NEW FRIENDS FILLED MY HEART
SHARING MADE FAST FRIENDS OF US

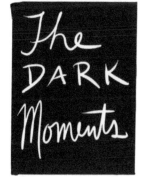 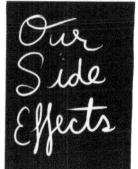 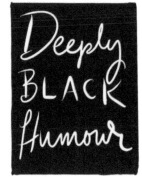

The DARK Moments

Our Side Effects

Deeply BLACK Humour

This is how we made eachother strong

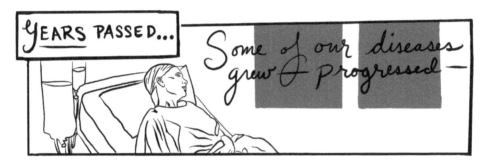

YEARS PASSED... Some of our diseases grew & progressed—

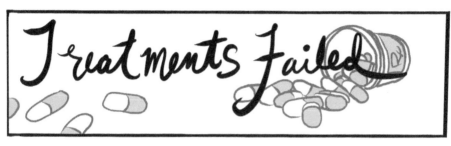

Treatments Failed

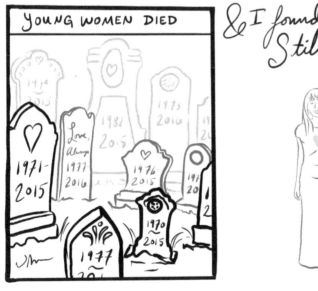

YOUNG WOMEN DIED

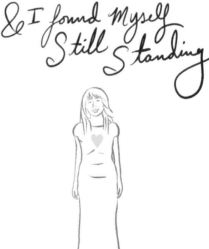

& I found Myself Still Standing

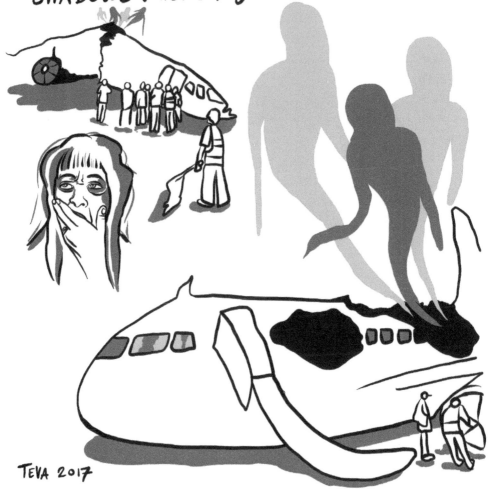

I FEEL DAZED — *lost* — LIKE I'M STUMBLING AWAY FROM A PLANE CRASH — *scraped &amp; bruised*, BUT <u>*alive*</u>, LOOKING INTO THE SHADOWS WHERE MY DEAD FRIENDS WERE

TEVA 2017

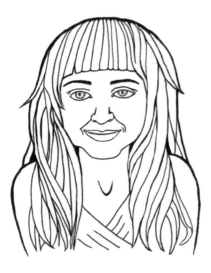

**Teva Harrison** was an artist, writer and cartoonist. She was the author of the best-selling graphic memoir *In-Between Days*, which was shortlisted for the Governor General's Literary Award for Non-Fiction, the Joe Shuster Award, and won the Kobo Emerging Writer Prize for Non-Fiction. She also created *The Joyful Living Colouring Book* and a posthumous collection of poetry and drawings, *Not One of These Poems is About You*. The drawings from *In-Between Days* were exhibited in a solo show at the Winnipeg Art Gallery, and she was also the lead illustrator on Jordan Tannahill's *Draw Me Close*, a National Theatre/National Film Board virtual reality theatrical experience. Teva wrote for *The Walrus*, *The Globe and Mail*, *Granta*, *Quill & Quire*, *Huffington Post*, and others, and was nominated for a National Magazine Award and a Canadian Magazine Award. She spoke widely on creativity, and led workshops on telling life stories. She was a strong advocate for people with chronic illnesses, and her works have been adopted into narrative medicine curricula worldwide. Prior to her diagnosis, she was the Director of Marketing at the Nature Conservancy of Canada, and before that worked in visual art, film, publishing and music. She was born in rural Oregon, and lived in Toronto with her husband. She died of metastatic breast cancer in April 2019.

Judith

Brain Drain.
Brain Trust.

John

Just another searing headache. It was bad enough to wake me at 5:00 am, and so severe it made me vomit. But that wasn't unusual.

The left side of my face felt numb and I suddenly had double-vision. But with two big presentations on my agenda, I could handle it.

Less than 24 hours later, I was admitted to hospital after doctors realized that my inoperable—but, mercifully, benign—brain tumour had haemorrhaged and was bleeding into my brain.

At the time, I just knew I was in terrible pain and had a busy day ahead. I took a handful of Advil and checked email. It didn't even occur to me that I should call a doctor, though I had several of them since being diagnosed with a pituitary adenoma 10 years earlier. I didn't consider calling in sick. I'm a strong woman, a professional, a mother. I don't complain. I push through.

*(But there are some things you can't push through. Like blood compressing the inside of your head.)*

We often think about trauma as abrupt, immediate, harsh: a blunt force, a car accident, a terrorist attack. *(Thank you, cable news and "Law & Order.")* But this was different. My inoperable brain tumour was stealthy and shifting, gradually changing me and my perspective from the day it was identified.

I've spent years ignoring brutal, long-lasting pain and discounting the repeated clues my body offered: a pattern of throbbing, worsening headaches; blurred vision, aching joints, lack of balance, dizziness, insomnia, extremes of hot and cold. I made myself think these were ordinary symptoms of a woman my age with a busy, stressful life. So I lived on painkillers, and bought stronger reading glasses. It's no wonder my daughter considers stoicism overrated, and often admonishes me with "Stoicism is Stupid."

Our culture celebrates strong women who are invincible, confident, and have it all, and all under control. Yet we punish ourselves for even admitting, let alone revealing, any frailty. In my case, it also had to do with my well-established family role, as the optimistic and positive problem-solver mediator middle sister. It's how I self-identify and how I was determined to present myself to the world, especially my children.

Yet, inside, I constantly deal with self-doubt, pain and guilt, despite having a loving family, amazing friends, and a remarkable, fulfilling career. Putting on a brave face can be especially hard, but that's how I cope. It was unthinkable that I would miss a day of work just because I was having trouble standing, seeing, and speaking.

So I went ahead successfully with the presentations—despite words and numbers blurring. It wasn't until a colleague noted I was ashen and my eyelid was drooping that I confessed, even to myself, that perhaps this was more than just an unusually severe siege of the recurring headaches. I was genuinely frightened that my time had actually come.

Fortunately, I was an executive at SickKids and my colleagues were doctors. As it's a children's hospital, the ophthalmologist, excited to examine her first mature eyes in years, peered into my brain. The reading was alarming: a big, grey lopsided bubble mass behind my eyes that sent me straight to a nearby adult hospital. At least there the gowns would fit.

It was a long night in Emergency, and I was now mortally afraid. I had lots of time to try to distract myself. I even did a fashion assessment. My bottom half was wearing the skirt of my business suit; on top, a hospital gown. My wedding ring was on my finger, and on my wrist, the plastic hospital bracelet. Such sartorial splendour.

I vividly relived all the nightmare scenarios I'd scripted years before, facing my first operation (through my nose, not through the side of my head) to remove the tumour. Then, with six weeks to wait for surgery, I wrote loving letters to my daughters for every occasion of their lives that I'd not be there to celebrate. That surgical attempt failed; those emotions remained.

The relentless pain and fear heightened my default to humour as protective armour. I unsuccessfully tried to convince the surgeon about to operate inside my brain to combine it with a facelift, but he had no packaging or marketing savvy.

Mostly I was reflecting that—however clichéd—life changes in an instant. It careens off the carefully constructed path, and leaves you wondering if there actually will be a next step, and where that might take you. In that moment, it's your response that defines you. What do you do when things go full-on catastrophic? Adversity rarely comes neatly packed as a single episode. It's a cascade. And despite optimism and experience, it confused and shocked me.

I didn't actually ask, "why me?" because I never considered this when life was smooth and wonderful. The real question, of course, was "why not me?" But I was terrified that I might lose everyone and everything I love, since I thought I'd die that night. If I survived, I resolved that while this was going to drastically change my life, it wasn't going to destroy it.

Miraculously, I made it through the emergency 10-hour craniotomy to remove the blood clots from my brain—and experienced a surge of profound, inexpressible gratitude. While the operation was a success—and I was alive!—the tumour's embedded location meant it could not be removed.

I faced a new and uncertain reality.

My surgeon pronounced my tumour inoperable, explaining we'd need to find other ways to deal with this active, stubborn mass growing in my head, that brought with it double-vision and the risk of stroke and blindness. The best treatment could only be determined as we watched and waited. I was forced to leave the job I adored, change my pace of life, and reflect on everything I took for granted. It was my "new normal."

With the chronic pain came an oppressive and lingering uncertainty. Physical pain has parameters and boundaries. Being sidelined in a state of limbo and no longer in control of my life was suffocating. Uncertainty about my very existence left me feeling adrift.

What I did have control over was my choices. I needed to reset my path and priorities. If work was the scaffolding of my previous life, I deliberately built a new one, seeking other ways to find meaning. I wanted to be a participant, not just a spectator. Aiming for grace and grit, not gold, I learned to be kinder to myself about my goals. More mundane accomplishments became my daily markers of success: walking a few blocks farther than before; concentrating enough to read a book instead of just skimming an article; volunteering.

My motto was right out of *Finding Nemo*: "just keep swimming."

My family was amazing. Strong, positive, loving, and connected. We continued to share lots of laughter. Admittedly, we do specialize in ironic, often black humour, which sustains us in almost any situation, from happy to grim (although it's a surprise to those who take things a bit more earnestly).

All kinds of people in my life helped keep me resilient, connected, and positive. While I have a healthy sense of openness and perspective, I remain keenly aware of life's randomness.

I still get blinding headaches, but without the fear that they indicate a stroke. The tumour itself is still there, despite two surgeries and the latest interventional radiology to contain its insidious growth. After an operation to tighten my eye muscles, I don't have to wear a patch, so I no longer look like a fashionable, middle-aged pirate. Though a friend did describe my look more evocative of "a cock-eyed optimist." I feel less uncertainty. Or at least more comfort embracing it.

I made some very deliberate life choices, because I was in charge of that.

I chose to move beyond my situation, not let it dominate or define me. I try to make it look easy. It isn't. I want to be a positive role model for my children. I hope they'll remember me as never giving up. And that, perhaps, they'll forgive my overdoses of enthusiasm. One of my daughters describes me (lovingly, I hope) as "the most stubbornly glad person, ever."

I try not to share pain (always fresh for me, tiresome for others) because I don't ever want pity or sympathy. I'm quite aware of how fortunate I am. I thrive on being engaged with the world issues and events, with my family (which now includes the joys of two grandchildren), friends and community. And that means nurturing vital human connections, always, no matter how I might feel at the moment.

And then, despite what I ironically called my "brain drain," came the serendipity that gave these dramatic changes to my life new meaning. I was asked to speak at a conference about my experience as a patient, since I'd had the unique privilege of looking at health care from three perspectives—as a hospital executive, as a long-term patient, and as caregiver for my husband, who was treated for cancer just as I was undergoing radiation to contain the tumour. All of this transformed my trauma into a catalyst that could actually help others.

Coupled with my career as a communicator and penchant for story-telling, these became a platform for advocating to improve the patient's experience. I saw how the healthcare system is designed around process, not people; metrics, not compassion. I felt first-hand how, for patients and their families, our healthcare providers have transformative power on every level, and that alienating disconnections happen because too often they forget the true basics: empathy, communications, and human contact. I learned that mutual respect and building trust are essential—

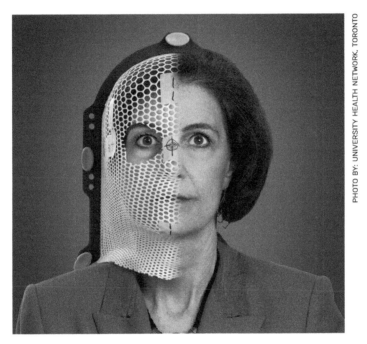

Judith John, with the radiation mask she wore each
day for six weeks, and with her recovering face.

that a patient needs to be treated like a person and a partner, not just a file number, an array of symptoms, or a diagnosis.

So I began speaking, writing, and training in order to help improve the healthcare experience for patients and their families. This mission has, perhaps selfishly, helped me make sense of, and peace with, all that has happened. It's inevitable and universal that all of us will become a patient or a caregiver eventually. As I've been privileged to speak around the world, it's clear that compassionate healthcare matters to everyone, everywhere.

The tumour actually became a catalyst to fill me with a new perspective, bringing unexpected opportunities and great people into my life. It taught me to make my relationships and my time really count. It reminds me—often painfully—of how beautiful and how fleeting life is. It remains a constant reminder to be grateful for so many gifts and new career pathways to live fully.

The trauma of brain drain has become brain trust—trust in myself, in others, in resilience.

I live as a fierce, incurable, serial optimist.

And, yes, I live with an incurable brain tumour.

———

**Judith John** served as Vice President of Communications and Public Affairs at the Hospital for Sick Children, and as Vice President of Communications and Marketing at Mount Sinai Hospital and Foundation. She is an international patient advocate, writer, coach and speaker about improving the patient experience, partnerships, ethics and communications. She has taught at universities across Ontario and has been a guest speaker worldwide, including at England's National Health Service and the first international Patient Experience Forum in Doha, Qatar. Currently she is Vice-President, Engagement and Marketing, for the Royal Ontario Museum Governors, a board member of the Michener Institute of Education at UHN, and sits on inter-institutional and government committees and panels, working to improve healthcare in Canada.

Jules Arita

# Intertwined: Speaking Our Truths

Koostachin

*In hopes of refuge*
*from her tears*
*I run*
*knowing I will never be free;*
*reaching for her, I fail to find her.*
*I dream once again*
*for the moment*
*she is free from her past ...*

As Indigenous people living on *Turtle Island*, we express ourselves from a specific Ancestral homeland, and from a socio-cultural location. I recognize that we each speak from our own distinct cultural values and principles, and as part of my protocol, I am expected to position myself prior to sharing my personal story.

I am *InNiNew*, a person from the Ancestral lands of the *MosKeKo*, and a band member of Attawapiskat First Nation, Treaty 9. I was born in 1972 on Moose Factory Island, found in what is now called northern Ontario. At birth, I was gifted with *MihKo WaaPiWin*, red eyes, which symbolize a person gifted with the ability to communicate with the spirit realm. I was born to an incredible woman named Rita, a strong *IsKwew*, a Cree woman who survived over a decade of imprisonment at the notorious Ste. Anne's residential school in Fort Albany, on the shores of James Bay.

My Ancestral name is *IsKwew MiSiMinKeWin IsKoTeo*, Women Who Holds Fire, and I am of the Bear clan. I am the granddaughter of Abraham and Zabeth. Abraham was an *OkiMawInNiNew*, a community elected leader of Lake River, a hunter and trapper. Zabeth was also a highly skilled hunter and trapper. My grandfather and grandmother only spoke *InNiNi-MoWin*, and I am a first-generation English speaker and urban person. I am the mother of four sons: *Asivak* (Spider), *MaHiiGan* (Wolf), *TapWeWin* (Truth Speaker), and *PaWaKen* (Dreamer), and I use media and other artistic platforms as a means to share stories.

My culture has taught me that we each define ourselves from a herstory—one that is woven within a collective memory, a memory that links the past to the present, and the present to the future. I am an Indigenous woman.

My existence has been both shaped and interrupted by my *InNiNeWak: people from the MoshKeKo*. I write against the backdrop of a life of working as an *InNiNew* storyteller in diverse fields of practice, and the knowledge and narrative I share is deeply placed within an intricately woven *InNiNeWak* belief system and reality.

I believe that our resilience as a people is determined by the strength of our cultural ways of knowing—otherwise understood as our sacred fires. My Elders remind me that our cultural ways of knowing, our sacred fires, were and continue to be sheltered and protected by our Knowledge Keepers, Elders, and our Ancestors. As a people, we strategize and resist; most significantly, we stay connected to the past, the present and the future through our ceremonies, relations, and through our relationship to our stories. Our stories keep us connected to our communities: the land, the water, our relations, and most importantly to ourselves.

> *Breaking open*
> *my heart heavy with hurt,*
> *I remember her.*
> *I remember her laughter*
> *her smile fills my heart*
> *with possibility.*

I understand what it means to experience intergenerational resilience. My grandparents encouraged me to honour our cultural knowledge systems as a means of survival, and without their influence my life would have gone down another pathway. As the daughter of a warrior, I have followed an exhilarating and necessary path of adversity, self-discovery and awareness. I have been forced to recognize how my mother's traumatic past continues to linger, interrupting our spiritual and emotional lives. I will keep saying these things. Keep seeing this truth.

*InNiNiMoWin* (Cree) is my mother's first language, and her broken English has made it difficult for her to communicate her story to us, her children. She made the choice to sever us from *InNiNiMoWin*, but I now know she was only trying to protect us from the racism she herself faced as an Indigenous woman. She tried hard to protect us, but it was hopeless. Even to this day, I can still recall her cries waking me up in the middle of the night. Hesitantly, I would go to her and lie beside her. Always face-to-face, I would look deep into her eyes, never knowing how to comfort her. I felt helpless as a little girl. I wanted to comfort her, but I was afraid to touch her. Her eyes vacant, her spirit would travel, leaving me with her emptiness. She would go back to her past. I lie there watching her remember. She looked through me, and then she whispered, her broken stories flowing. Her stories were a mix of English and *InNiNiMoWin*. Her stories were always so disconnected, yet horrifying. After what felt like an eternity, her spirit would find its way back to her body. Suddenly, something would snap inside her, a battle. Just being beside her triggered her, and then, her anger. There I was trapped, helpless lying there with her, afraid to move. It was as though she was angry for my bearing witness to her stories, like I had done something horribly wrong. Her voice, loud and annoyed, would shame me and send me away again. All I wanted was to make her feel better, and my presence seemed to make things worse for her, and for me.

My brothers and I, although raised in *InNiNiMoWin* during the first years of our lives, were moved south because my mother was seeking employment. In Ottawa, my mother made the choice to only speak English to us, alienating us from our *InNiNiNeWak* family and community. Despite her sacrificial efforts, we were still exposed to racism. When I was five years of age we had just moved to a new low-income housing project. I was struggling with hearing loss due to severe ear infections, so I was very quiet and shy with new people. When school finally started, my mother would walk my brother and me to school in the morning. I was terrified because it was all so different—new school meant unfamiliar people. For a few weeks after my mother dropped me off, I would quickly sneak away from class, chasing after my mother. I did not want to be left there with my teacher. She was tall, masculine and her hair was a white short bob. Her sour face was yellow with age; deep lines ran across her forehead. She never smiled, always scowled.

Thinking back, it is remarkable to me that at a young age, I sensed that she did not approve of my family. At the time, I was confused as to why she had animosity towards us, but I would soon find out. After several weeks, and many escape attempts, I finally built up the courage to speak to a little girl in my class. I remember asking her to play with me at recess. She smiled back at me, and my heart warmed. I was so proud of myself for reaching out. I was excited to make friends because I had been so lonely. Suddenly, my teacher approached me, and proceeded to call me a *savage* in front of my classmates. *What is savage?* Then, she raised her hand and hit me hard across my face. My small body flew back, and confused, I looked up at her unsure of what I had done. My face welted up, and it was sore to touch. On that day I learned to be silent, and sadly, I also understood that in order to survive in school, I had to disappear. When I saw my mother later that day, she asked me what had happened and I told her. Instead of being angry, she seemed worried. I saw fear in her eyes. My mother dropped me off at school the next morning with her head hung low and handed me over to the teacher without addressing the assault. I understood I was alone, and she would not protect me. Today, I understand that my mother's lack of response was a symptom of her own institutional abuse—she had spent her childhood being treated that way. *Why should it be any different for her children?*

*Silence*
*Loathing the feelings imprisoned inside her*
*Possessing her soul*
*Wintiko—Cannibal Spirit*
*She wanted to set it free*

My mother resisted the temptation to remain silent. Her frustrations grew and she became progressively angry with herself and with us, her children. She struggled to find the right words to articulate her feelings, and when she finally found the courage to share, it came out fragmented and worn. My mother would speak of men and women with pale eyes dressed in black cloaks who took Native children out of their beds late at night. She would speak of zombie-like children returning to the dormitories paralyzed in fear; silently crying themselves back to sleep. Children were not allowed to speak to their siblings, and they were beaten for speaking their language. Children were locked up when they misbehaved, which meant acting like an *Indian*. She spoke of children woken up early in the morning to work, cleaning up after the nuns and priests. My mother would say that the children were always cold and starving. There was no laughter, just silent tears echoing throughout the building. The most horrifying stories were of the children that died there, and never returned to their families. She told me that their families would wait for their children's return, but nothing. Nothingness ... Silence ... Pain ... Suffering ... They hated us for being Indian ... Hungry ... Evil men ... Evil women ... Darkness ... Silence ... Nothingness ...

Being on the receiving end of her stories was often confusing. I was puzzled, unsure how to respond, because her stories were disturbing, and I hate to admit, they were preposterous. Her stories were filled with suffering and pain, darkness and horrendous child abuse. My young mind could not fathom how she survived her experiences, and I was perplexed as to why the nuns and priests would intentionally hurt children, especially when they claimed to be religious. It made no sense to me. *How could you say you are religious, a person serving God, when you hurt children? God was supposed to be kind and loving.* Nothing my mother told me was making any sense, and I knew in my heart that something awful had happened to her when she was small. *Why else would she tell me these stories?*

I found myself furious at my mother's anger towards us, it seemed that her anger only fuelled my rage. My siblings and I were helpless as we struggled to relate to her. She was overwhelmed by her childhood memories, and as a child I remember feeling robbed of a mother. I recall thinking that mothers should be kind-hearted, affectionate, and loving, yet my mother was always irate, depressed, aggravated. As a child I was fearful of her, and afraid to reach out to her; for the most part as I got older I remained silent, or hidden away from her. There were times when she laughed, a bellowing belly laugh, and when I heard this rare laughter my heart filled with joy. Her happiness filled my world with light, and her laughter helped kept my spirit awake.

> *Her anger pushed us deep inside ourselves;*
> *broken trust prevailed.*
> *Dreaming of her love*
> *holding on to what could have been.*

In 2008, the Canadian government finally admitted to the cultural genocide of Indigenous peoples. Although the apology was controversial to many people, I believe it was necessary to start the process of healing. I was a student at the Summer Intensive Film Program at Ryerson University. The day of the apology remains vivid in my mind. I excused myself from class a few minutes before the scheduled apology. I headed toward the Chinese restaurant across the street and asked the owner if I could watch the apology on his television. He happily obliged, so there I was in a Chinese restaurant watching the news, alone.

I stood there crying as I listened to the Prime Minister of Canada publicly acknowledged my mother's stories. My heart was heavy. *Those ghastly and unbelievable stories I grew up hearing were true. They must be true if the Prime Minister is apologizing.* To be clear, I did not need the apology to believe her. It is a hard emotion to articulate. I was overwhelmed with a sense of relief, grief, shame and guilt. I had spent so much of my youth frustrated with her for pushing me away, and all she needed was my love. *Was I a bad daughter?*

Speaking to this experience is challenging, my feelings are difficult to express. My best attempt to share my feelings of the apology is in one word: *accountability*. The apology was much bigger than an affirmation. Perhaps it was more about the state's accountability to my mother, and countless others who suffered at the hands of violent perpetrators.

I remember feeling that the weight I had carried with me my whole life had been lifted from my shoulders, and that the deafening silence was breaking. I wiped away my tears, and headed back to class. As I walked across the street I noticed that nothing had changed. People were walking about as though nothing had happened. That day will be fixed in my heart forever.

Since the apology, I have witnessed my mother struggle as she navigated her way toward culturally appropriate counseling and through the court system. I helped my mother with her legal paperwork, and helped prepare her for her testimonies. I was beside her as she provided the judicator an uncensored version of her story, stories she had carefully sheltered me from. Stories of how she survived the abuse she endured when held captive. Her stories of neglect, sexual and physical abuse, are forever engrained in my mind. Now as an adult, I understand that these are her stories to tell, and that although I have been deeply impacted by them, the stories are for her to share and on her own time. I also acknowledge that it took her sixty years to finally work up the courage to testify against her perpetrators, and therefore I need to be respectful of her healing process.

I sat there helplessly, my stomach turned inside out, and I felt stabbing in my gut. The heaviness of hearing the abuse she suffered slowly suffocated me. Something shattered inside me, and a new form of rage surfaced. I was always her voice, she called upon me to speak for her, and here, suddenly, she was speaking for herself. Her courageous, resilient and strong voice finally breaking free. She was speaking out against her abusers. *What is my role now? She won't need me anymore?* Something remarkable happened. Through sharing our stories, counseling and ceremony we have carefully put the pieces of her story back together. As a mother myself, I have learned the importance of facing our fears, letting go of what is holding us back and the healing powers of speaking our truths. *What is my truth, now that she released hers?*

While travelling on my own healing journey, I have had to rely on my culture and ceremonies as ways to reconcile with intergenerational trauma. I have had to define reconciliation for myself, and work toward my own healing, to make certain my children are free from the emotional and spiritual burden of the residential school experience. Each and every day is a challenge, but it is my children who provide my spirit the hope to face the day. I share with them my story and it is through story that I have been able to articulate my own truth. My Elders taught me that the *truth* lives in *spirit*, and our *spirit* lives in the stories we choose to share, and that the words living within our stories may hold the medicine we require to move beyond our own pain. Our stories have the capacity to unite, create change, raise consciousness, and heal. There are times when the stories are trapped inside the inner parts of ourselves, and we have become accustomed to keeping them protected. We protect ourselves from reliving the pain when we keep them deep inside; it's a survival mechanism. *How do I separate the pain from who I am if it's always been there?*

When sharing my own experiences of trauma I am faced with the weight of my own humility and fear. Overwhelmed, I find myself afraid to confront the demons. My mother's story has become mine, intertwined and inseparable. I can no longer tell where her story begins and mine ends—perhaps that is the way it has always been. Our stories of resilience have become one, and the pain we shared continues to connect us. My mother braved the stripping of her *self*—each layer of her *being* stripped away by the continuous abuse against her spirit, body, mind, and heart. After a decade at residential school, she was left in disarray and unsure as to who she was as an Indigenous woman. She tells me that she became trapped by fear, self-hate and depression. She was stuck by her inability to share her story, her life became too painful to live, and her future too agonizing to dream. She dealt with each day the best she could, and it is because of our culture that she is with us today.

To this day, we continue to heal as a family, and I am sure it will take time to fully comprehend what has transpired. My mother is my hero; her strength drives me to be a better mother, and a better person. It is through the experience of being her daughter that I have come to realize that I too matter. My *voice* is important, and my stories also matter, especially to my family and my community. Our silence has been broken and finally set free, and it was my mother who broke it with her words.

*Heavy heart*
*Spirit starved*
*Mind fragmented*
*Dreams broken*
*Breathing*
*Resilience*
*In knowing our roots.*

My cultural teachings have allowed me to find my way back to myself. Our life experiences shape our stories, and as hosts, we are responsible to the story. Our stories provide a pathway back to our *spirit*, which is the ultimate connection to our relations, the land, water, and to our Ancestors. *All my relations*. Our stories provide the pathway home.

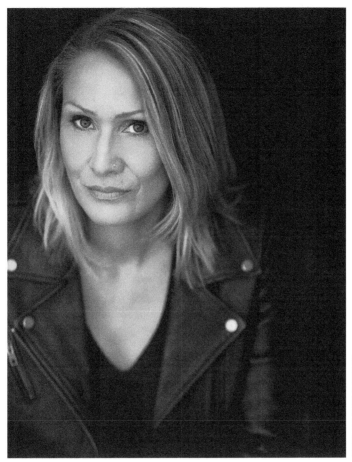

PHOTO BY: KAROLINA TUREK

**Jules Arita Koostachin** is a Cree filmmaker, writer, actor, activist and a proud mother of four sons. She has several publications of poetry, short plays, and book reviews, and is currently working on a collection entitled *Children of the Survivors: Intergenerational Resilience and Canadian Residential Schools* with the University of Regina Press. Her films, installations, television series, and documentaries focus on Indigenous culture, both rural and urban. She has extensive knowledge of the arts, and works as an instructor at several institutions. Jules is currently completing her PhD at the University of British Columbia with the Institute of Gender, Race, Sexuality and Social Justice.

Alison

# The
# Old Me,
# The
# New Me

Langham

I woke up one morning in August of 1995 with my forehead, cheeks and temples screaming. My ears were ringing. I couldn't open my mouth. The pain came from within me, within my skin, within my bones. Worse, I didn't know what had happened between the preceding lazy summer night when I fell asleep and eight hours later when I woke up.

Thus began my life with temporomandibular joint jaw disorder (TMJ). I spent the next 20 years coping with daily headaches, an inability to chew, and sometimes problems just speaking, yawning or sneezing—all of which comes from a displaced and deformed jaw joint.

After multiple surgeries and treatments, I was resigned to the fact that chronic pain was a part of me. This was the *thing* that would define me and shape me. No explanation. No warning. It just was. And yet I always thought I would defeat it, triumph over it. I thought of myself as strong and inspirational, and I took pride in the strength of mind over matter. I hadn't let this chronic condition negatively take over my life. So, it was to be my thing, my defining thing. Right? Wrong.

On November 17, 2011, my husband, our beloved hound, and I were cruising west on the 401, to meet Toronto friends for dinner, followed by yet another jaw surgery the next morning. At one point just outside Trenton, our car, like all the others, had to stop for construction. A typical, almost predictable stop on the 401. Nothing special. Just a bit frustrating.

I didn't see, I don't remember the 10-tonne semi-trailer truck tearing down the hill behind us, while we sat stationary, stuck. I don't remember our compact car crumbling into a distorted mass of metal and plastic, wedging itself into the front of the semi, and bowling vehicles out of the path in front of us. I don't remember the sounds. I don't remember the flames that engulfed our car and the motorists who extracted us from the wreckage and lay us on the the road, amidst the carnage.

Lights flashed around me as I lay on my back staring up into the faces of strangers: a cluster of hovering masks. The masks flashed on and off in sequence with the emergency lights. My next memory was being lifted from the ambulance gurney onto the emergency room bed and hearing the clinking of broken glass that was sprinkled through the blanket, reminding me of the chaos.

Blood dribbled through my hair and down the back of my neck. I felt nothing as the wound was stapled 28 times. My right foot that had jammed under the gas pedal was swollen and it was painful to swallow. Aside from multiple bruising inside and out, I was okay. I do remember, clearly, the doctor expressing his amazement that I had survived such a catastrophic accident.

I read about the accident on the Trentonian website:

**UPDATE: Fatal Collision on Hwy. 401 near Trenton**

At least one person is dead following a serious multi-vehicle crash on Hwy. 401.

The six-vehicle accident occurred around 3:20 p.m. Thursday on the westbound lanes of the highway near the Glen Miller Road in Trenton.

Constable Christine Quenneville, media relations officer for the OPP, reports that one person has been killed, another victim, transported from the scene by air ambulance, sustained serious, life-threatening injuries.

One vehicle caught fire.

Traffic came to a complete halt in both directions due to scattered debris. The accident involved one tractor trailer, which was carrying a load of dates which scattered onto the highway.

One vehicle involved has also been identified as a Corrections Canada van which was carrying one inmate, who sustained minor injuries.

OPP officers are also reporting several minor, separate collisions on the westbound highway lanes due to vehicle drivers not paying attention in heavy traffic and due to traffic slowing down.

The days after the accident were a blur. I was confused and scared. But alive. People shook their heads in disbelief when they saw the pictures and heard the news stories. My husband, hound and I had made it through.

We should count our blessings and appreciate our "good luck," right? I still looked the same. I hadn't lost any limbs. I was unconscious throughout most of the ordeal so wouldn't even have horrible nightmares of the actual event.

The days and weeks that followed included multiple tests that were requested by my family doctor.

I was lonely, even though I was surrounded by friends and family.

I was happiest in my bed, where I could lay motionless. One of the concussion symptoms was pain associated with light. When the sun shone upon me, I would get an excruciating headache. When there were gloomy clouds blanketing the sky, I got severe headaches from the glare.

Because I was so fragile, emotionally and physically, my physiotherapist sent me to a swimming pool as a way to soften my journey back to normal life. For weeks, I became a buoy in the pool, bobbing up and down, the only thing I was able to do. In the echoing, Olympic-sized pool I began to realize how much I had changed. Each morning, I watched the senior's water aerobics class at the other end of the pool, thinking "I am half their age, and all I can do is watch their class."

It was the simple things that frustrated me. Memory loss. I was not only forgetting things, but was anxious about what I might be forgetting at any given moment. I wasn't prepared for a head injury that left me unable to remember the PIN number on my credit card and being unable to recall what I ate the previous day for dinner.

The unpredictability of my emotions occurred at the flip of a coin. I could switch from laughing to crying, feeling patient to angry, with no warning to myself or others.

Because I could only filter one sound at a time, I rudely overreacted to people around me. In my mind, I felt perfectly justified to react with frustration. The sounds I was hearing made no sense. And then my anger was followed by embarrassment and regret. I could no longer cook a meal all at once but had to perform one single task at a time. I found myself fading in and out of conversations, got headaches from lights and sounds, and felt I had to suck up the humility and disappointment that came from all this.

And then the self-doubt and sadness.

At first, I fought the idea of getting to know (and accept) the new me. Most certainly the old Ali wouldn't cry for no reason, or get dizzy while walking up stairs, or get so anxious that she often couldn't eat. It became a battle between the old and the new me. How easy it was for me, before the accident, to imagine how my life would have been.

My competitive edge had been lost.

Why set goals if they were unattainable?

I would be excited to meet friends for a meal, and knew that I needed them, and that I wanted to reconnect with them. But with other sounds—voices from another table, background music—I could not understand the conversation around me. I would panic, get embarrassed, and start to cry. I began to wonder if there was any point at all in trying to socialize.

I used to jog 5 km quite easily. Now I got dizzy from simple movements.

I used to enjoy parties. Now my husband and I had to pre-plan the social environment I would be in. Sometimes my husband would go without me, or we would plan to drop in to an event and then leave right away.

I used to spend lots of time on the computer. Now I couldn't face the screen for longer than 15 minutes before I got a headache that lasted for hours.

I used to work and contribute towards our household income. It was now almost impossible to find any type of work that could accommodate my limitations.

One day, my psychologist told me that it would be a lot easier if I learned to accept the new me. I told her that I didn't like the new me, I didn't like my new invisible disabilities. Her response was to question how I knew that I didn't like the new me since I hadn't given myself a fair chance.

No one's journey is pre-scripted. We don't get to dictate what obstacles, challenges and experiences confront us.

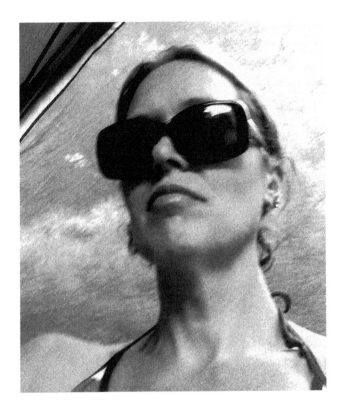

In time, I have learned that those familiar parts of myself that I loved and developed before the accident remain in my core, my spirit. They are a part of me that will never change. But I also realize that I cannot be inspired and hopeful and excited about my future.

I don't truly know and accept the new me. My new self.

No one can anticipate or prepare themselves for that split second of time that changes the world forever. There may be more than one of these moments in our lifetime. My *thing* is not one single major life event that I must overcome, not one ordeal that I learn from, which in exchange entitles me to a free pass for every other bit of sadness or trauma that I would have had to face. It's a combination of lessons, losses, pain and jubilation that are markers in teaching me all of the gifts that I have.

We are resilient creatures. The underlying human need to love and be loved, and to be hopeful of the future, remains a strong motivator.

Did my chronic jaw pain help to prepare me for the head injury and changes that were written into my story? I don't know. I like to believe that it did, but maybe it doesn't matter. I now have a titanium jaw joint that helps me enjoy my new favourite dinner, steak.

That's a small thing.

———

**Alison Langham** is an entrepreneur at heart. She managed a unique boutique selling imported Middle Eastern and Asian home décor and furnishings for eight years. She also enjoyed operating a seasonable kitchen tools kiosk. She looks forward to initiating a new business venture in the future, but her current job is recovering. Among other therapies, her pets provide snuggles and companionship that are indispensable. Residing with her, just north of Kingston, Ontario, is her amazing husband, Dan, who reminds her that, at the core, she is the same woman that he married 18 years ago. She still loves pigging out on popcorn and enjoys gardening, exercising, and reading. Sometime in the future, Alison aspires to return to volunteering at both the Kingston Humane Society and Big Brothers Big Sisters of Canada.

Valerie

# No One
# Said the
# D-word

McDonald

Our gentle oncologist told us what we already knew, that our seven-year-old daughter, Natalie, had Acute Lymphoblastic Leukemia or ALL. The diagnosis, she said, was upsetting, but the good news was that 80 percent of children like her were cured. That meant that 20 percent died.

A dozen people, mostly women, sat with us around the conference table in the hospital's windowless room. The table was littered with papers, and cups from Tim Hortons. My husband, Bruce, kept notes, jotted names and asked questions. I spent the disclosure meeting wiping tears and wondering how I could live without my lively, artistic middle daughter. I wondered what effect her death would have on her two sisters—Maddie, who struggled with learning disabilities but regarded Natalie as her best friend, and four-year-old Anna, who pretended she didn't, but truly did worship her older sister.

No one said the D-word.

Over the next weeks, Natalie's physicians and nurses patiently repeated the information I hadn't consciously heard at the meeting. They taught me about treatment protocols and blood counts and re-introduced the members of our team. There were nurses and social workers and child life specialists and a psychologist who conducted baseline neuropsychological testing. We learned to be grateful for the phlebotomy team and a purple-haired clown named Posy. Everyone was upbeat and positive and everyone made an effort to put Natalie into the 80 percent category. I quickly mastered the rules of our new cancer culture: Be positive, focus on cure, and never say the D-word.

The treatment went badly at first. Natalie developed infections in her central venous lines, became diabetic on prednisone and needed daily insulin shots in addition to chemo. Her grandmother tried to help by paying Natalie a dollar a needle but we asked her to stop when the tally reached three hundred dollars in eight weeks. We spent nearly six months in hospital during the first, most intense phase of her treatment, and then the 80 percent goal blazed into view. Natalie's infections cleared up, the prednisone was tapered and her blood sugar returned to normal. At last, she was in remission.

I patted myself on the back about my positive attitude, my attempts to help Natalie "visualize" herself defeating her leukemia blasts, and I was immensely grateful that we lived so close to the best children's hospital in the world. We spent a glorious hot summer at the cottage and took our three girls camping on Georgian Bay. Natalie learned to build a campfire, had diving contests with her best friend Annie, and stayed up late to spot shooting stars. She went back to school in the fall and jazzed up her wispy new hair with ribbons, certain that her trademark strawberry blond hair would soon be restored to its disheveled glory.

In December, in the middle of a baby shower we were throwing for my sister, Natalie called me to her bedroom. "Something's wrong," she said, and showed me her underwear soaked in blood. I tried to be calm and think of reasons why an eight year old might start menstruating early. But a few days later, on Christmas Eve, we had another disclosure meeting. After two years of chemotherapy and radiation, Natalie's cancer had relapsed.

Research has found that parents' recognition that their child had no realistic chance of cure lagged behind their physicians' understanding by more than three months. Contrary to this research, my understanding matched that of our physicians. I had never stopped worrying that my daughter might die. But because no one said the D-word out loud, I didn't either—at least not to the staff.

My friend Lori summed up our attitude. Her two-year-old daughter Chloe had been in hospital for half her life and Lori knew she was going to die, although she didn't believe it. "But I don't let them know that I know," she said, "Otherwise, they'll give up on her." During the day, Lori challenged her doctors with findings from articles she read to double-check Chloe's treatment. But at night, when we met in the tiny parent kitchen, she told me about funeral plans and wept.

Like Lori, I was afraid the staff would give up on Natalie, so I didn't use the D-word. The research says that when physicians and parents both recognize that children have no realistic chance of cure, there is a stronger emphasis on treatments to lessen suffering.

After the relapse, we were offered two options: an experimental chemo that might put Natalie into remission long enough to have a bone marrow transplant or "no treatment." We chose treatment. No one talked about how to lessen her suffering.

After Natalie relapsed I noticed that some of the staff had started to avoid us. At first I thought I was being overly sensitive but one day our whole family stood together in the busy clinic waiting for Natalie's blood work. Nurses and doctors who had known us for two years passed by without acknowledging us or even seeming to see us. "Wow, now I really know how Harry Potter feels under his invisibility cloak," Bruce said.

I understood how difficult it must be for the staff to know that their efforts hadn't worked, but I felt isolated and scared. Much later, one of the nurses who had avoided us confided that she hadn't spoken because she didn't want to upset us by talking about Natalie's impending death.

One person did speak to us about death. Shortly after Natalie relapsed, the psychologist came by. She knew we had received bad news and although she sincerely hoped that Natalie would get better, she wanted to tell me about the kinds of concerns that dying children typically have—just in case the treatment didn't work.

She used the words *die* and *death*.

I was furious but she persisted. She told me that dying children worry that they will be in pain, that they will be forgotten and that their families will not be okay after they are dead. I sat with my arms folded, glaring at her without speaking or asking any questions, but I remembered every word.

The treatment was brutal and it didn't work. Natalie's new, wispy hair fell out and she developed a fungal infection that made her big toe turn black and die. Plans were being made to amputate it when the infection cleared up, but by then she acquired a pink wheelchair that her sisters loved to push.

This time, our gentle oncologist used the D-word. She told us that Natalie "probably would die," and suggested a regime of palliative chemo to "give her more time." Only then did we discuss ways to relieve her suffering, enhance the quality of her remaining days, and help her die.

I never gave up hope that she would recover.

We decided that we wanted to be at home when Natalie died so that she could spend time with her sisters, visit her friends, sleep with her cat, and get to know her new baby cousin. We told Natalie that the leukemia had come back.

We didn't use the D-word.

Before we left the hospital, we had another team meeting. This time, I knew that everyone at the table would help me in any way they could. I wanted to know how Natalie would die, when she would die, how I could help her die, and how I could help Maddie and Anna. But I didn't ask any of those questions. I didn't want to believe that I needed the answers. And because I didn't ask, no one offered any guidance. Instead, we talked about ordering supplies and made lists of who to call if we ran into problems at home.

At home, everyone was happier. School was over for the summer and we spent lots of time on the front porch, reading, visiting with friends and playing with my sister's new baby. The kids took turns racing the pink wheelchair with Natalie—and each other—up and down the block. Natalie spent hours drawing and working on crafts. She taught herself to make beaded animals and bracelets, giving all her creations to her sisters and friends.

One afternoon, as I sat reading to Natalie in her bedroom, she asked, "Mom, am I going to die?"

Because of my meeting with the psychologist, I knew I had to tell her the truth.

"Yes, Natalie, you are probably going to die."

"When?"

I fought back tears. "No one knows for sure. I hope it will be a long time from now."

"Will I be able to be a flower girl in Uncle Dave's wedding?"

I thought of the lace dress that my future sister-in-law had chosen for Natalie and I knew she would not wear it at the wedding. "I really hope so."

"What will happen to my money and all my stuff?"

I laughed. Natalie's grandmother had paid the full $300 of needle-money with a bag of loonies. "You can decide what to do with your money," I said. "As for your stuff, we'll keep your drawings and art work forever and ever. But if you want to give away anything special, you can decide."

Then she said, "What happens to me?"

I didn't know what to say. I'd stopped believing in anything remotely like Heaven that might offer comfort. But I reminded her of a conversation

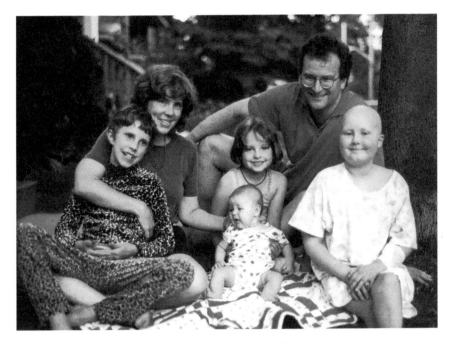

Photo taken just before Natalie died. Me, my husband,
and our three girls with my sister's new baby.

I'd had with my mother before she died. "You remember what Nana said. She said she was going to a place where it's always warm and there are lots of flowers. You'll be with Nana."

She didn't want to talk anymore. A few days later, I asked her if she wanted to make decisions about her money or giving away her favourite belongings.

"No," she said, "I don't want to decide yet because we don't know *when* I'm going to die."

Not long after, Natalie died at home in my arms. In her last moments, she struggled for breath. I said, "Natalie, you don't have to fight any more. Nana is waiting for you. You should go with her now. I'll love you forever and ever."

Her body relaxed and her face was calmer and more peaceful than it had been for many months. She looked well again.

And then she was gone.

When her paediatrician came shortly afterwards to pronounce her death, I stood by him as he gently examined her. I was certain he would tell me that she was just asleep.

I simply could not believe it then—and I still don't today—that my Natalie had died.

Trained as a social worker, **Valerie McDonald** is a freelance writer and editor who also serves as a patient/caregiver representative on the pan-Canadian Oncology Drug Review committee. Her articles and short stories have been published in *TESL Talk, Storyteller Magazine, Paperplates, Hospital Quarterly* and *Canadian Stories.* Valerie leads a feisty writing group known as The Bathurst Muses and is currently working on young adult novel.

Rocky

# My Sister Tina, the Strong One

It was 20 July 1969. Man walked on the moon. It was the earliest significant historic event I remember. We watched it unfold on the late night news, my father explaining it to me as I gazed at the moon in the dark sky. I was only four, and my baby sister, Tina, only four days before her second birthday, was dragging herself along the floor on her tummy. That's how Tina moved around. I did not think much about it at that time, but over the next few years my family would have to accept the harsh reality that Tina would never walk.

Nobody could explain it. She was a "perfectly healthy" baby. She pulled herself up as a one-year-old, holding on to a fence in the garden, a fleeting moment captured by my older sister on her camera, a photo that my family would cherish forever. By the age of two she could sit up, play with toys and drag herself along the floor, but she could not stand. Over the next year her mobility and dexterity worsened and soon she could no longer feed herself. She could still sit up in her high chair, but even that became difficult.

After countless medical consultations it was determined that Tina had a developmental neurological disorder. It never seemed clear exactly what was "wrong." Nor did it matter what doctors said. I remember words like "cerebral palsy," "crippled" and "mentally retarded." My parents and two older sisters struggled to understand and accept this. They visited "alternative" practitioners, some more akin to "witch" doctors, trying various remedies, hopeful that something might work. But nothing made a difference.

It was only after Tina started attending a "special school" did I start to fully understand the challenges she would face in her life. I remember the day when the wheelchair arrived. It was sleek and shiny. It felt as if she was getting her first bike, but my brief moment of excitement soon turned to sorrow as I saw my mother holding back some tears as my dad brought the chair into the house.

The social worker helped us get the wheelchair. She was an older lady who visited every few months. We would sit at the dining room table and my parents would sometimes struggle to understand her. And I remember the brochures about the "institutions" that she left behind one time, and how my mother put them in the bottom drawer of her night table right after she left.

Tina's condition continued to slowly deteriorate until the age of 16. By this time she was essentially a non-verbal quadriplegic, confined to a wheelchair and requiring dedicated care for all her daily living functions. At this same time I was graduating high school, top of my class, and about to enter university on a full scholarship. I worked hard, but things came easy for me. I was grateful for my good fortune—I had freedom, independence and many other things that Tina did not—but it felt I had been granted these privileges at her expense.

My two older sisters had young, healthy families; they worked hard and succeeded in business. I followed many years later, started my career, was married and blessed with a beautiful family of my own. All the while my parents devoted themselves to providing loving care for Tina throughout her lifetime, with unrelenting dedication and determination. The level of care that Tina required became increasingly demanding, and as my parents aged they became less able to provide. They struggled to overcome many, often very difficult, challenges. But it was a labour of love and in return Tina filled our lives with joy and many wonderful memories that will be cherished forever.

Tina died a few months before her 40th birthday, shortly after being admitted to hospital for a seizure, and due to complications from pneumonia. Her passing away came as a sudden and devastating jolt to everyone.

Measured in years her time with us was too short, but measured by the amount of people she touched it was a long and special life. Tina enlightened the lives of so many people in so many different ways. She was always the heart of the family—she was the focal point, and often the light of the party. Whether it was a small gathering at home, a family outing, or a birthday party, Tina had a way of making it special for all those who were in her presence.

To those who knew Tina in the community, at school or at her day program, she was the quiet, cheerful young lady who enjoyed socializing and being part of the crowd. Tina did this in her own unassuming and modest way, and always with a smile on her face. She did not have extravagant needs and took great pleasure in the simplest of things: a quiet conversation, going for a stroll in the park, enjoying a cup of coffee, or listening to

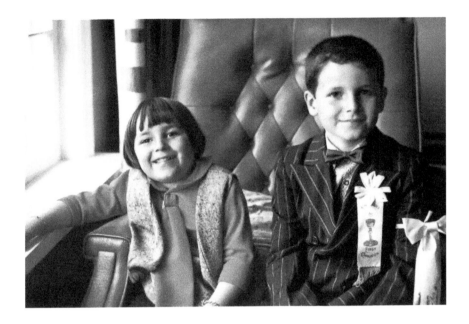

music. All one had to do to make Tina happy was to hold her hand—she needed only to be loved.

My relationship with her shaped who I was as a young man; she provided me a frame of reference, an anchor, a flag post in the ground—something that defined where I came from, where I was, and where I was going. When God took her away He took part of me, too, and I felt lost without her, my sense of direction seemed distorted, unclear. I was too afraid to admit this, even to myself, because I felt the need to be strong as she had always seemed so weak. I did not tell her often enough how much I loved her, and there remains in my heart a cavity full of regret, for which I have asked God for forgiveness, but that will always afflict me to some degree.

I know why God chose Tina to be saddled with so many challenges, instead of me. I would not have survived because I was the one who was weak, not Tina. God gave me a healthy body and perhaps a good mind, but he gave her the purest of spirits and a boundless ability to trust and love and express her emotions—things which I lacked.

Although man was able to walk on the moon, Tina was not able to walk a single step in her life. Yet hers was a journey that most of us would not have the courage to travel. She had the strength and determination to overcome her physical limitations and the many obstacles she faced as a result. She was an inspiration to everyone that knew her, and her spirit remains with us forever.

––––––

**Rocky Morra** was born, raised, and educated in Toronto, is married with three sons and resides in Port Credit, Ontario. A professional engineer by trade, Rocky has spent the majority of his career at Microsoft empowering people and organizations through the adoption of software to improve their day-to-day lives in meaningful ways. He also enjoys classical music, reading, and volunteering in his local community.

Marina

# The
# Chemistry
# Notebook

Nemat

I put my Toyota RAV4 in reverse and pulled out of the driveway. On my quiet street in the suburbs of Toronto the mature maple trees provided some shade, and the white domes of hydrangeas—too heavy for their long, thin stems—touched the grass, surrendering to the humid heat. The neighbour's sprinkler sprayed golden droplets into the air.

On the main road, traffic was light. People were on holidays, splashing in cool northern lakes, sipping iced tea and beer on the docks of cottages. I tried to keep my focus on driving. The traffic light changed from green to amber; I stopped and felt my breathing. In and out. In and out. After the railroad tracks, I merged onto the highway, and the landscape of farms dotted with new subdivisions became a blur.

I had not seen Mitra in 35 years. Would I recognize her after all this time? We had been 16 years old back then, children really. Now our kids were in their twenties. Would she be mad at me for all that I had and had not done?

A few months earlier, she had found me on Facebook after the publication of my memoir, *Prisoner of Tehran*. When I saw her first message, I stared at her name as if I had received a letter from Mars. The black letters on the white screen tattooed themselves onto my soul.

She had found me.

"Do you remember me?" her message read.

Perhaps it was possible to forget my family, even myself, but I would never forget my cellmates. Never. In the early 1980s, we had been teenage prisoners of conscience in Evin prison in Tehran. I had been arrested because of speaking out against the new religious laws that came into place soon after the Islamic revolution in 1979.

After a 35-year gap, Mitra wrote that she was coming to Canada from Iran, where she still lived, for a family visit. She wanted to get together. The weeks since she first contacted me felt like being on a spaceship, trying to reach another galaxy that might not even exist.

The evening I received the news of Mitra's visit, at the dinner table, I told my husband, Andre, about her plans.

"Wow. After all this time. It will be interesting," he said and put a meatball in his mouth.

*Interesting?* That was one way of putting it.

I nodded, keeping my eyes on my plate, forking the spaghetti drenched in garlicky tomato sauce.

"You excited?" Andre asked.

"Yeah."

My voice carried a tremble that was too subtle for him to notice. The meaning of this meeting was enormous. No emotion was capable of containing it. I didn't want to betray what I felt with words. Andre had not been in Evin. No outsider could ever understand.

"Would you like more meatballs?" I asked Andre, and smiled.

I almost missed my exit off the highway and had to break a little harder than I liked. With a quick check of the rearview mirror, I decided it was safe to change lanes. A white cloud shaped like an enormous fish floated in the neon-blue sky. In Evin, we watched the clouds when we were allowed to use the courtyard, surrounded by the brick building of our cellblock. We imagined that clouds could take our messages to our families. Barred windows of public cells—each housing between 50 and 70 young women and girls—punctuated the two-storey walls. Armed guards—all male—kept watch over us from the rooftop, so we had to wear the complete Islamic hijab while outside. For exercise, we walked in a circle, as if around an invisible nucleus. We were fragile, strong little planets of sadness, floating in a space that light would never enter. In our space, the sun of freedom had died.

In the heart of downtown Toronto, I slowed the car and found the entrance to underground public parking close to Mitra's hotel. The cool, cavernous space calmed my nerves a little. I found a spot and backed in. Then I checked my reflection in my small mirror: my eyes had dark circles around them. My heart raced. My legs felt heavy as I stepped out of the car.

The street buzzed with pedestrians rushing, cars honking, and bicycles weaving in and out of traffic. Even though I could see and hear my surroundings, a strange but familiar distance had wedged itself between the world and me. I entered the foyer of the hotel. Travellers with colourful suitcases rushed past faded artificial plants, and suit-clad hotel workers with forced smiles on their tired faces greeted guests at the counters.

Elevators dinged. The smell of sweat mixed with the scent of air fresheners. I stopped on a floral rug in the centre of the foyer and searched the faces of passersby.

"Mitra, where are you?"

My eyes caught her as she exited an elevator. She had cut her hair short, very short, but she looked the same except for a few wrinkles on her forehead and around her eyes. Her face was as pale and serious as I remembered. Her piercing dark eyes met mine, and she smiled. We embraced.

This was a place beyond grief. We held each other in the middle of the oblivious chaos. For a few moments we had a small but safe space to acknowledge the pain that we each carried. Tears were inadequate and superficial. We stood at the edge of the memory of mass graves. I could hear the gunshots of the executions that ended my cellmates' lives, and I was sure Mitra could hear them, too.

She took my hand and guided me to a quiet area of the lobby where there were a couple of empty couches. We sank into one of them.

"Marina..." she whispered.

My name meant something different when she said it. It was the name of the young girl I had been, the one who had died in Evin. Mitra's voice summoned that girl back to life. She gave birth to memories, making them real. The past became the present. We were 16 again.

"What did you do after you were released?" I asked.

We had both been in Evin for about two years, but we had never been in the same cellblock.

"I did nothing for a while. Then I studied at home and got my high school diploma. Then I wrote the entrance exam to enter university. My marks were close to perfect, but universities didn't accept me because of my prison record. But I didn't give up. I kept trying. After four years, my parents bribed a few officials, and I got in. I became an electrical engineer."

We talked about our families, especially our kids, until I found the courage to ask what I really needed to know. During my tenth grade, 1980-81, I had been very outspoken, protesting the government's attack on the rights of women and freedom of expression. In the spring of 1981, toward the end of the school year, when the mass arrests of young people began, I had a nervous breakdown. That was when I decided to take time off school—I didn't attend eleventh grade.

"What happened to Shahnoush?" I asked.

Shahnoush Behzadi had been our classmate and mutual friend.

"She was executed," Mitra said, her voice a whisper.

"I know, but when?"

"Late November 1981."

"I was arrested in January 1982."

"I was arrested a few days after Shahnoush."

"Why did they take you? You weren't very outspoken in school."

"It had to do with Shahnoush."

"How?"

Mitra played with her wedding ring. Her left eye twitched.

"In summer 1981," she said, "Shahnoush asked for my chemistry notes and I gave her my notebook. She came to my house and picked it up. She said she'd give it back to me on the first day of school, but on the first day she wasn't there. When she didn't show up on the second day, I called her house, and a man I didn't recognize answered the phone. I asked if I could speak with Shahnoush. He said she wasn't there. I asked when she'd be back. He said he didn't know. I told him that she had my notebook, and I needed it back. He told me to go over to the house, and he'd give it to me. The way he talked made me nervous, so I hung up. That night, the Revolutionary Guard came to my house and arrested me. The man I had talked to on the phone was a member of the Guard. He was at Shahnoush's house, searching it, and he answered the phone when I called. Shahnoush's older brother was shot and killed when the guards went to their house to arrest them. Shahnoush's phone was being tapped, and they found my address. When they were interrogating me in Evin, they thought that 'notebook' was a code name for something else, something important. They beat me to a pulp..."

Mitra had been arrested for a chemistry notebook. I should have become accustomed to such scenarios, but I was still surprised at how something so small and simple could lead to so much suffering.

"They beat me, too," I said. "They lashed the soles of my feet. After what seemed like eternity, I couldn't take it anymore. I signed every document they gave me without reading them. They wanted the whereabouts of a young woman, a friend of a friend of mine. She was a university student, and I didn't know where she was. I would have told if I knew. They already had a list of names of 'anti-revolutionaries' from our school; our principal had reported us to the Courts of Islamic Justice... What was the principal's name? Khanoom Mohammadi or Mahmoodi? I can never remember..."

Mitra nodded. Her eyes followed a few teenagers laughing as they passed us.

"Shahnoush and me were in the same cellblock for a while," she said, "the one they called the Apartments. They kept calling her for interrogation and beating her. She was talking back to them. I told her not to. They gave her a death sentence..."

"I had a death sentence, but I lived, because I broke, because I gave in when they threatened my family..."

"Would it have helped anyone if they had executed you, too?"

"She was 15..."

"You were 16."

"She should have lived. She was better than me..."

"She was better than both of us, but she died. Marina, you have a gift, you have a voice, and you can use it. I live in Iran, so I can't say anything. You've written a book about what happened to us. They can't erase that. Your book will live on. Thousands of people have read it, and many more will. You've done what most of us can't. You live in a free country, and you can use your voice. You have to make sure that Shahnoush won't be forgotten. Promise me!"

She took my hands in hers and squeezed them tight, her eyes pleading. We couldn't reach into death and bring Shahnoush back, but we could keep her memory alive.

I wanted to become a medical doctor when I was growing up in Iran. Then Evin happened, and for years, I remained in an emotional coma, unable to feel much. I began to show symptoms of Post Traumatic Stress Disorder and had a major nervous breakdown in 2000. To deal with it, I wrote and wrote, and my writings became *Prisoner of Tehran*. I hoped that once I published the story, I would heal, that the pain would go away, but it didn't.

I discovered that there was no such thing as closure; I could not "close" the past and bury it. Being a witness to mass murder and crimes against humanity could never be a part-time job; it demanded everything I had.

Mitra and I talked and talked. After we said goodbye, I watched her disappear into the elevator. I thought that would be the last time I would ever see her. But our bond was stronger than place and time: it wove us into one. I would keep my promise to make sure that our memories would survive, even though many of us had not.

———

**Marina Nemat** was born in 1965 in Tehran, Iran. After the Islamic Revolution of 1979, she was arrested at the age of 16 and spent more than two years in Evin, a political prison in Tehran, where she was tortured and came very close to execution. She came to Canada in 1991 and has called it home ever since. Her memoir *Prisoner of Tehran* was published in Canada by Penguin Canada in 2007, has been published in 28 other countries. In 2007, Marina received the inaugural Human Dignity Award from the European Parliament and, in 2008, the Grinzane Prize in Italy. She was the recipient of the Morris Abram Human Rights Award from UN Watch in Geneva in 2014. She is the chair of Writers in Exile at PEN Canada and teaches creative writing at the School of Continuing Studies at University of Toronto.

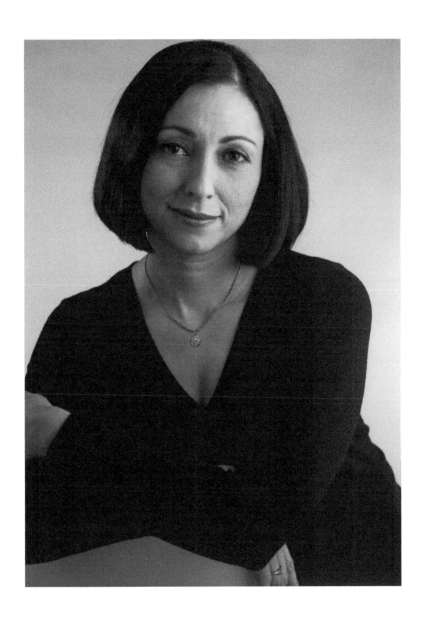

Peter

# Walking
# Shadows

O'Brien

In May 1959, a family photograph was taken on our front yard in Mamaroneck, New York, not too far from Winged Foot Golf Course, one of the most storied and elegant private clubs in the U.S. It is a bright day. Ten children are dressed up and squinting into the sun, with a mother and father loosely bracket the randomness. My sister Lauralee holds a doll, and Bridget holds two stuffed animals. Brothers Bob and Ed are wearing matching suits. My mother is on the left side, holding my younger sister Patty, two months old and wailing, and my father is on the other side, holding me, the second youngest. The strap of my suspenders has fallen off my right shoulder and I am grabbing for it, oblivious to the photographer's task.

The black and white image captures all the joys of the passing moment: my dad's white pocket square and shining shoes, my mom's cat-eye glasses and the smiling pleasure of her expanding world, with the trees and the columned porch as a stately backdrop. My dad, working for an international airline company, is wrapping up a five-year stint in New York, preparing to move us all to Rome for the next five years.

Perhaps this photograph was taken to preserve the memories of our last spring in the U.S., or to introduce my father and his voluminous family to the new world we were to be a part of in Italy.

Two months later, my dad went for a routine medical check-up. The doctor decided to run a few more tests, this time in a hospital. Some concerns about a flutter near the heart.

My dad never came out of the hospital. He didn't make it to 50.

I don't remember the details of his hospital stay, his death, or the funeral. I don't remember my mother packing up her ten children, or the five days we spent on the train heading west to Vancouver, where my mother started her life again, amid her brothers and sisters and her aging parents.

I have been told that my mom was incredibly strong through her final days in New York and as she set up her family for our new life at the other edge of the continent. And then, when she had done what she needed to do, she collapsed into the blind sadness and harsh absence that I'm sure consumed her. I don't remember her climbing out of her widowed grief to get on with her life. I do remember as a boy visiting her at Joan's Fashions, the humble dress shop where she worked on 41st Street in Kerrisdale. I'm not really sure how she found the strength or the time to work at a dress shop and to make sure we kids had what we needed. Joan's Fashions—with its dark and cramped interior, and its colourful splashes of patterned wool and polyester draped over hangers lining the walls—is long gone.

I don't know what led my mom, a few years later, to marry a widower and add 12 stepchildren to her family. I do know that she always found space in her heart for whatever was asked or required. My maternal grandfather—cantankerous and testy—lived with us until he died, chastising and scolding us with snippets of Oliver Goldsmith's "The Deserted Village." Uncle Fred, my mom's twin brother—covered from head to toe with psoriasis from the trauma he went through during WW II—lived with us for a time. Flakes of his skin ... un-melting snow ... dusted all the surfaces in the house. My Aunt Alma—blind and with Down Syndrome—also lived with us until she died. I see her still, walking from room to room, her arms outstretched, touching the walls with her fingertips, finding her way.

Somehow my mother's house expanded to meet these various needs. "Of course you can live with us. For as long as you want. We have lots of room." That's the sort of thing my mom would have said.

Our lives are built upon these additions, these absences. The passing people, the deaths. We fill our lives with conversations, and entertainments, and activities, but the foundation of it all is people who have died and memories that have faded.

My brother Bob, suited and smiling in that 1959 photograph, was 12 when my dad died. He was a rambunctious teen, a willing soldier in Vietnam (as a Canadian, he had joined the U.S. army to be "part of the team," as he told me many years later), and a loving father to his son and daughter. But he also had demons. When he committed suicide it was a shock that reverberated throughout the family. Unthinkable. Impossible to understand. Perhaps inevitable. No one saw it coming, although the seeds must have been planted many years before. A slow, relentless germination.

For each of us, the largest part of the record of our family no longer exists: all of the multitudinous adventures and tribulations, the tears and smiles of the fleeting centuries. Fractured stories of homes left behind, dissembling families, vanishing histories.

We carry the absences with us. There's nowhere else for them to go.

I only have one thing from my father. It's a small oblong pine box. On the side of it, my dad wrote in black felt pen:

To Pete   From Dad   1958   Hong Kong

He must have picked it up on one of his frequent overseas trips. Inside, there are 31 members of a musical band: blobs of painted clay stuck onto wire legs inserted into the wooden surface. Some of the band members play tiny yellow flutes and others beat small drums. Two carry flags, stiff little swaths of gold and red cloth. Two ride horses, one reddish-brown and the other white.

The leader of this tiny, silent band is missing—there is only a small bent wire where his body once was.

I don't remember my dad giving this gift to me and I don't remember playing with it as a child. I don't know how the body of the band-leader disappeared.

There is a story of this gift—of the person in Hong Kong who made it, painting with tiny brushes the eyes and the mouths on each clay figure; of my father buying it for me; of my mom putting it away for me—but the entire story has to be fabricated from missing details.

The only way to tell the reality of this story is to make it up.

Soon after my dad died a good friend of his was finishing off a book. Elmer Wheeler, known as "America's Number One Public Speaker," had already published 21 books: a range of travel and diet and sales books (he was the person who coined the now ubiquitous phrase "Don't Sell the Steak—Sell the Sizzle"). Elmer's new book, *Around the World with Elmer ... Backwards*, is a jaunty travel book subtitled *How to Haggle in 17 Countries*. Known for his "girth as well as his mirth," Elmer writes about various international adventures, including a Tokyo burlesque show, a "Sultan's Harem" in Turkey, and "How to Drink 27 Foods in Beirut."

My dad is referenced several times in the book. He had suggested to Elmer to make sure he got a hair cut in Hong Kong. "It's a world beater," says my dad, "one you won't forget." Elmer refers to my dad as "Lee of New York."

In the "Forewarning" to the book, Elmer writes about a visit to Merida, Yucatan, "whose ancestors date back nine centuries." Describing the women and men of Merida, he says: "I can't explain my feeling ... Look at the newsboys. Look at the shoeshine boys. Look at those store keepers: all are sitting quietly, almost as if they knew Death, the Great Reaper, was on the way, yet none seem to care."

The book came out in 1960 and is dedicated to my dad:

To

Lee O'Brien

Who has made his "last flight"

over the horizon.

I have the copy that Elmer gave to my mom, which he signed in black felt pen:

To Mrs. Lee O'Brien

A 1st Edition to a 1st Edition

Tucked into the book is a letter that Elmer wrote to my mom, dated October 27, 1959, on his personal letterhead from the "Sizzle Ranch, Dallas Texas: Where the East Peters Out." Elmer tells my mom that all the mentions of Lee will remain just as they were originally written, and ends the letter with the words "Lee, indeed, was a good friend of mine. I'll always remember him."

Of course Elmer is now long gone. As is his memory of my dad.

Sometimes stories, like people, meander around, get lost, distracted. Sometimes they die.

I didn't spend five years of my childhood in Rome. I didn't get to ask my dad for his advice or opinion. I don't remember him telling me stories.

I'll always remember him, but it's only through temporary, disappearing things: a black and white photograph, and an oblong wooden box that encloses a small, soundless musical band with a wire where the leader used to be.

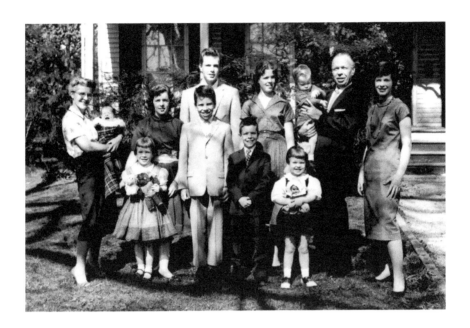

**Peter O'Brien** has written or edited seven books, including *Introduction to Literature: British, American, Canadian* (Harper & Row) and *Cleopatra at the Breakfast Table: Why I Studied Latin With My Teenager and How I Discovered the Daughterland* (Quattro). He has published articles, reviews, and artwork in *The Globe and Mail*, *Montreal Gazette*, *Art / Research International*, *The Fortnightly Review*, and *World Literature Today*. He has worked as a ladies shoe salesman, a roughneck on oil rigs, a professional fundraiser, an environmental entrepreneur, and in corporate communications. He was a founding Board member of White Ribbon, the world's largest movement of men and boys working to end violence against women and girls.

Eric

# "Daddy, what's this?"

Petersiel

I have spent the past week sleeping on the floor at Toronto's Hospital for Sick Children, praying that someday in the future I'll be able to tell this story to my now one-month-old daughter.

She was four years old the first time she asked me, "Daddy, what's this?" pointing to the three-inch hockey stick forever inscribed beneath her ribs.

"A scar, from an old boo-boo," I replied. And that was enough. For then.

When she was six, the scar was barely a pencil-line of pigment-free skin running for an inch below the top of her yellow-polka-dotted bikini. "You had surgery when you were two weeks old," I told her. "They took out a bad thing that was inside you and then you were fine."

At age 14, it was barely visible, a fold of skin on the smooth complexion of her oft-revealed midriff. But the more insignificant the evidence, the more pressing was her need for further explanation. She was leaning on my shoulder as we watched college basketball on a lazy Sunday afternoon, her long dark hair draped over my shoulder. She was tall and skinny, with her mother's angular chin. Although she was still a little awkward, it was clear to me that she would someday be the most beautiful woman I would ever know, just as I considered her to be the most beautiful baby, child and teen before that.

"I slept on the floor of the hospital for a week the month you were born. It was the hardest week of my life." There is no way I could ever explain to her all that her mother and I felt that week—how it changed our lives and our relationships forever, but it seemed that the time had come to try. "The day after you were born, ultrasound tests showed a growth just above your kidney and we took you to the hospital the next week to have it removed."

The vast majority of adults who live with a solitary kidney have no knowledge of the fact. But halfway through the gestation period a pre-natal ultrasound alerted us to this oddity in our daughter. At each step of the way the healthcare professionals make it clear: "This is not a huge deal. She will be a normal child. These things are somewhat common."

Following the joy of labour and delivery, my exaltation was tempered by the calm paediatrician who did the initial examination. "There are a couple of little things, no big deal, which you should know. These here," he said, pointing to the previously unnoticed extra pinky fingers on each of my daughter's hands, "they take them off in a few weeks. The plastic surgeon will be through to look at them and describe the procedure. Very common, nothing to be concerned about."

One in 500, say the statistics. Filipino culture considers a sixth finger good luck, and leaves it be, but our society can't handle difference too well, and I simply couldn't face my little girl knowing I could have avoided some of the ridicule she would face. Advantageous, perhaps, in kindergarten counting exercises, until the smart-ass average simpletons with the perfect teeth and the blond hair make her the brunt of their jokes in the fifth grade, making her (and by extension me as the person responsible for her deformity) miserable.

"And this here," the young physician cooed, "this foot is not really a club foot, just not quite stretched out properly. The orthopaedic surgeon will be in to talk about correcting it later."

What are you talking about, I thought to myself. What the hell could be wrong next with this kid? My answer came the next day.

"On day two of your life," I told my daughter, "the paediatrician told us that a CAT scan would be required to clarify something odd they had found." An ultrasound, which measures blood flow, had picked up a blood-flowing mass in her abdomen which was neither her solitary kidney nor one of her two adrenal glands (which secrete hormones into the body, including steroids to monitor blood pressure, hormones to calm stress, and helps to even out the balance of electrolytes).

Our child just kept getting more special. One in 100,000 babies is born with a neuroblastoma, and still it is considered the most common of tumours identified in babies. Only 50 percent survive, a statistic fortunately not relayed to me at the time.

"I cried when they took you for that CAT scan. They stripped you down, stuck an IV into your arm and strapped you to the table so they could take pictures inside you. The nurse taking out the IV had a little trouble and you sprayed blood everywhere. When they handed you back to me, they told me not to be afraid if you looked like you had been in a war-zone."

Not to be afraid of her blood sprayed all over the floor of the lab on her second day of life? I was petrified.

"The doctor explained to us that the growth seemed to be a neuroblastoma, and we would have to check you in to The Hospital for Sick Children. The condition simply wasn't common enough to be fully understood in the hospital where you were born."

"How are you doing? Are you tired?" Everyone asked me for weeks after you were born.

I spent the second night of my daughter's life with her passed out on my chest, imagining the worst. At one point I simply assumed that my baby was not meant to survive. That all of the factors added up to an unhealthy baby who didn't deserve to live beyond the morning. And if we could simply get on with it ... she would die ... and her mother and I could leave the hospital to start again on creating a family. I never breathed these words aloud, but my delirium after 48 hours awake, and the wall of negative information flooding my brain, found this to be a calming and comfortable solution.

I never over-interpreted to include religious justification, or accepted this as divine retribution for some past misdeed. I simply accepted that she was not meant to live. I record those thoughts here only because I am so sickened that they crossed my mind and know that they can never be uttered aloud.

"I know I left the hospital much grayer than when I entered, thanks to you," I poked her.

"On your second Tuesday of life we checked into the hospital. We were just getting used to having you home, to splitting the duties of rocking you to sleep, catching naps when you were asleep, diligently charting your feeding schedule and the frequency and quality of your pee and poop. We held you for the last few hours until we handed you to the nurse to take you into surgery. It was 8:00 in the morning and your mother and I held you together as we cried. Handing you off was the hardest thing I have ever done."

What if that was the last chance I had to see her? Was it fair that she would have lived in this world for two weeks only? By the time we spent our first night at home I had abandoned my horrible thoughts from the hospital and wanted more than anything in the world to never let her go. I meant it literally. I did not want to hand my baby over to that nurse to disappear behind those doors for five hours of drugging, slicing, bleeding, removing and stitching.

I looked around the waiting room and tried to understand the feelings of those around me. Some had clearly been there before, their children already active participants in chemotherapy or looking somewhat disfigured in wheelchairs. For the whole week I judged people by the looks in their eyes. What was the prognosis with which they were dealing? Had they been told that their trial was "common," and that success was high? How many were told to consider failure?

The first waiting room was for surgery. After a week in hospital, I got into the habit of checking it out each day. By 8:00 am during the week, three or four families were camped out on the pleasant looking pastel blue and yellow couches, having been checked in by the efficient volunteers, always white women over the age of 60. I thought about them having to spend their days in the monotony, explaining to each family where the free coffee was, where the bathroom was, and writing down their identifying features so they could be corralled quickly upon arrival of some news from behind the closed doors of the surgical suites. We waited five hours in that room. A number of families spent an hour or two. Some families must have been struck with horrendous news, but it was never clear to me. The volunteers kept their cool, and chatted with each other about recipes or the theatre as the day dimmed.

Some days I noticed a family there all day. By 10:00 pm—with the volunteers gone, the cafeteria closed and the free coffee vanished—they waited for a word on the health of their children.

On the weekend there was no surgery booked. The room had no volunteers and no coffee. The odd family, uninformed, uninstructed, unfamiliar with the experience, waited for someone to tell them how it had all gone. I wanted to reach out to them. It had taken less than a week for me to feel like a true citizen of the hospital, weaving my way through the ins and outs of living in the place, not as a patient nor an employee, but a prisoner in a 10' X 12' cell with free reign over the grounds at any time of day or night.

"Following the surgery you were moved to the Critical Care Unit, because your blood pressure had dropped and they had to stabilise it with drugs and give you blood." What was that like on the inside of the

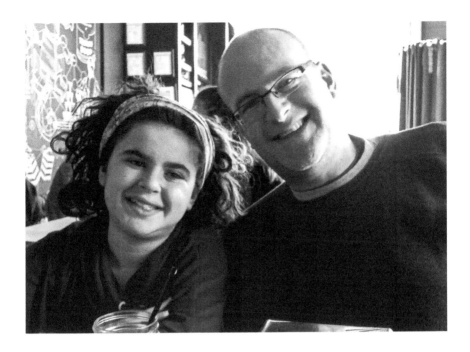

operating theatre? Were they screaming at each other to stitch her up, to find the leak, to jab her with extra drugs like an episode of ER?

The CCU waiting room was brutal. No volunteers, coffee, bright pastel couches or staff. I learned quickly that the state of the CCU waiting room was based on the state of its clientele. We lived there for two days, greeting visitors from the niche we had carved out for ourselves in the corner by the fish tank, and walking in with them to see our daughter, sedated and full of tubes. Parents and grandparents lived on the couches day and night, some for weeks on end.

Two-year-old Nadia came over to us to point out the fish she liked. We met her parents, and heard that they had been living in their corner of the room for six weeks as they prayed for the health of Nadia's sister, two months old. We exchanged niceties with them, offering Nadia a cookie or using her pretty smile to lighten up the conversation. At the end of our week, I didn't have the guts to go back down to see how they were.

"You spent your final three days in a private room. Your mother slept on a bench and I took the floor. We celebrated the smallest things: the first time we were allowed to hold you, the first time you breastfed after three days without food, and the beautiful moment they removed the last two tubes and we got to hold you. We both cried and fought over who would get to hold you longer. Neither of us wanted to ever let you go. We came home, and you recovered, beautifully, which is why this has never been an issue we had to discuss with you."

**Eric Petersiel** is head of The Leo Baeck Day School, the largest Reform Jewish elementary school in North America, and is certified by the Reform movement as a Reform Jewish educator. In 2005, he and his wife Tami Moscoe started Lilah's Fund, a registered family fund at the Hospital for Sick Children in Toronto. The fund directs financial support to research aimed at developing more effective and less harmful treatments for neuroblastoma patients.

Ed

# The
# Tangled
# Garden

Pien

In 2004, during a research trip to China, a small paper-cut caught my attention. It was a crudely rendered symmetrical depiction of a head suspended in the top centre of a tree, with two figures facing the trunk below. It was childlike, yet mysteriously powerful, and I imagined it alluding to magic or some long-forgotten rites. It also reminded me of an engraving made by French artist Jacques Callot called "La Pendaison" or "The Hanging" (from "Les misères et les malheurs de la guerre," 1633), which depicts a disquieting scene where a multitude of bodies hang dead or dying from a giant tree. I am not entirely sure what it is about trees that allure me and why they are recurring motifs in my paper-cuts, but they speak to me of childhood adventure, of birth and death, and of fear and the unknown. Struck by what I saw in China, I started working with images of figures in trees. I began to make paper-cuts because I am interested in paper as a medium and am also captivated by the silhouetted form. I decided to create these works large-scale to rival painting, and to counter the quaintness or preciousness generally associated with this technique.

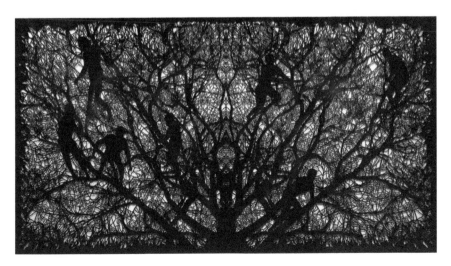

**Night Gathering**
2005, ink on hand-cut Shoji paper, 243.84 × 487.62 cm

163

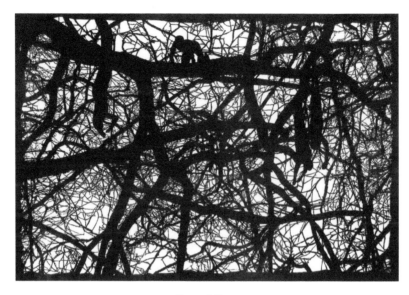

**Sacred Tree**
2007, ink on hand-cut Shoji paper, 396×259 cm

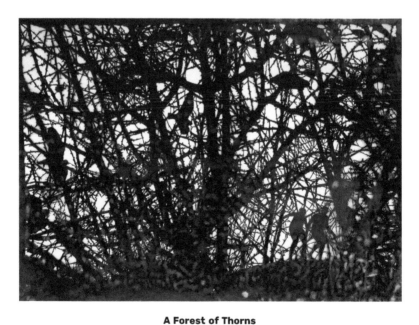

**A Forest of Thorns**
2007, ink on hand-cut 3M reflector film laminated on Shoji paper, 182.88×134.62 cm

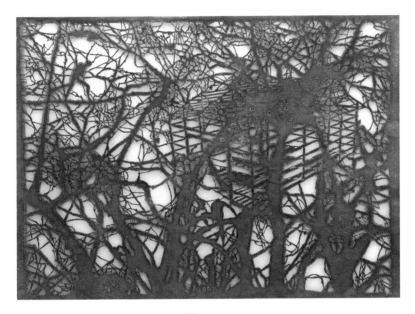

**Unscape**
2008, hand-cut 3M reflector film laminated on Shoji paper, 123×92 cm

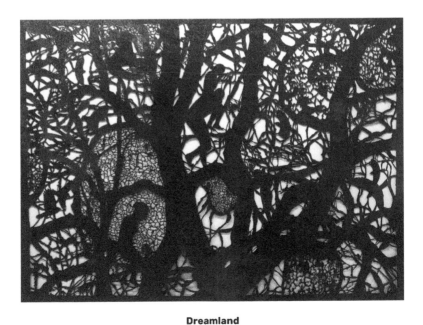

**Dreamland**
2010, ink on hand-cut 3M reflector film laminated on Shoji paper 182.88×134.62 cm

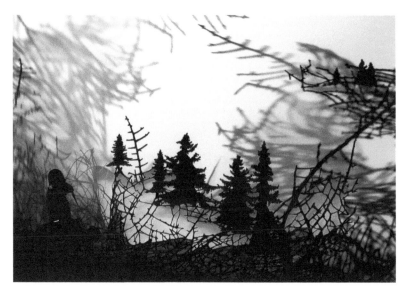

**Crawl**
2010, cut digital print, 116.84 x 77.75 cm

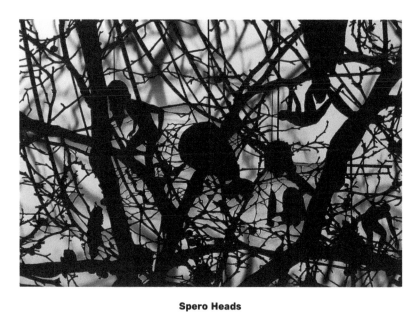

**Spero Heads**
2010, cut digital print, 116.84 x 77.75 cm

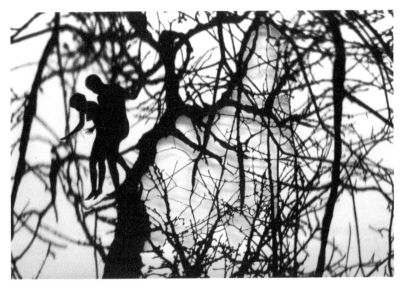

**Untitled**
2010, hand-cut digital print, 116.84×77.75 cm

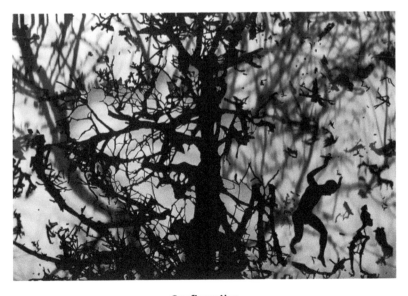

**Conflagration**
2010, hand-cut digital print, 116.84×77.75 cm

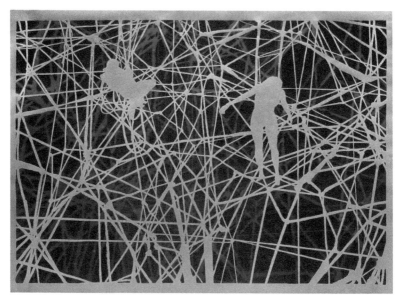

**Suspend**
2012, hand-cut 3M reflector film laminated on Shoji paper
layered over ink on Shoji paper 121.9 x 91.5 cm

**Ed Pien** is a Canadian artist based in Toronto. Born in Taipei, Taiwan, he immigrated to Canada with his family at age 11. He holds an MFA from York University and a BFA from Western University. Pien has exhibited nationally and internationally, including in the Drawing Centre; the Victoria & Albert Museum; The Goethe Institute, Berlin; The Art Gallery of Ontario; Musée des beaux arts; Musée d'art contemporain; Oboro, Montreal; The Mendel Art Gallery, Saskatoon; Songzhuang Art Centre, Beijing; the National Art Gallery of Canada; and MASS MoCA. He has participated in the Montreal Biennale, the Sydney Biennale, and the Moscow Biennale. He teaches part-time at the University of Toronto. Pien is represented by Birch Contemporary in Toronto, Pierre-François Ouellette Art Contemporain in Montreal, and Galerie Maurits van de Laar in The Hague.

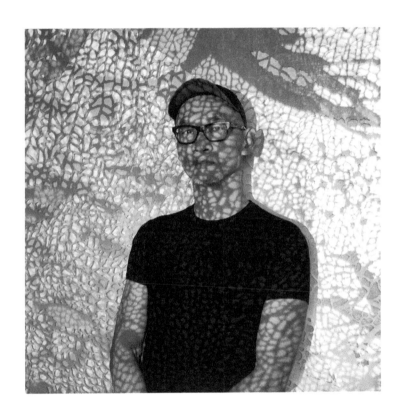

Neena

# Navigating
# My Darkness

Saloya

I am Neena Saloya.

I have been blind since birth.

Both my brothers were born in New Delhi, India. They died many years before I was born. One brother lived for several hours—he was unable to receive needed surgery—and my other brother was miscarried.

I was born in Toronto in 1974. I have lived most of my life in Canada, with two extended trips to India: for nine months when I was six years old, and for three months when I was 12.

Both my parents died before I reached the age of 30. My parents had a restaurant for 17 years and my father was also a chef in several hotels. He had come from India to Montreal to work at Expo 67 and my mother moved to Canada to be with him in 1972.

I try not to be overwhelmed and saddened by people who do not see who I really am and do not see the good things I have to offer.

My father and mother always believed that I would find a "big job," although my mother was always more supportive of me. She paid for me to further my education. She also tried to help me lose weight by encouraging me to do an exercise where I would spin my torso and move my arms.

My mother regularly took me out to eat, up to the week before she died. The last memory I have of her was wanting to go on a walkathon. I didn't go, because that would have meant missing the last lunch I had with my mother.

My favourite memory of my father is when he came out of the hospital, after being sick, and he would guide me. We laughed together, up to the day before he went into a coma.

When I was 21 he said to me, in his native Hindi: "Neena, it's amazing that you're sitting here knitting, and talking with me, while you listen to music. Other girls your age would have been fooling around or doing other things. You're quite accomplished, child."

My parents' ancestry is Jewish, although my immediate family did not know this heritage. My ancestors were expelled from Spain after the Spanish Inquisition. They moved to India, thinking they could work there and practice their faith. In India, my family was forced to adopt Hinduism. People say that this happened eight generations ago.

I recently finished my master's degree and I give credit to my faith in the divine to be able to function at all! I am a Jewish person with Seventh Day Adventist leanings.

Not being able to see is a disadvantage, but that makes me want the world to be even more accessible to people with disabilities, the marginalized, and the poor.

The strength that is inside me threatens sighted people, because I stand up for myself. They think about how they treat blind people and their guide dogs. It also threatens other blind people, because I won't just accept their words the way they want me to.

To keep going is tough. To circumvent the darkness of peoples' attitudes, and go out with my guide dog is often an ordeal, and involves a lot of planning. Even going out to buy dog food can sometimes turn into a three-hour event. For me, that means needing to depend on others for basic needs: "can you help me find bread?"; "can you show me where the bathroom is?"; "can you point me toward the subway?" There are days when I think that it is just too much.

It can be hard to fit in to a world where almost everything is built for sighted people.

I hate not having braille labels on public washroom doors!

I want to be able to go where I want, without having to ask a sighted person where a washroom is, or a coat rack, or a specific room I'm looking for. The more I have to ask sighted people questions, the more they feel they can comment on my life.

Sighted people often do not regard blind people as equals. At a store I was asked by a lady of my own South Asian culture: "Don't you have family to help you? Why don't you have someone to help you right now?"

I was frustrated and angry: "I don't have family! I don't have friends galore who I can ask to break up their life's wants, and help me!"

I have to strain and push like a woman giving birth to an over-sized child to fit in to the demands of a sighted world! People have gotten upset with me for not using a fork to eat fries, or because I have dog hair on my dark shirt, or I have a stain on my blouse.

Do sighted people ever try to fit in to a blind person's world? No! Sighted people sometimes have bad days, but I am told: "Forgive, forget, and move on!" I'm not able to have my own "bad day" without hearing angry replies from sighted people over the silliest exchanges!

Shop clerks and others sometimes try to sway my purchases and dissuade me from things I really like. Once, I wanted a blouse. A former instructor of mine threatened me that she would never take me shopping again if I didn't buy a certain dress. She said it looked wonderful on me. I kept craving that blouse. Well, I washed that dress once too often, and now it is unwearable. I resented this person, and finally just told her not to be my instructor anymore.

God forbid if I kick up a fuss. Everyone around always reprimands me. As the blind person, am I supposed to "put up and shut up," and "be grateful for small mercies that people want to throw at me?!"

I scream a silent mutiny and say: "No!"

There are other good times when I do go out with my guide dog, Fargo. We get a lot done on those days. We meet wonderful grocery clerks that help guide us around stores. These people love how my dog guides me to the counter. I love going to my two favourite restaurants and feel them accepting my guide dog and me.

But there is a sinister thing that haunts me and bites me unexpectedly. It is the throbbing pain of betrayal, compounded by uncertainty and grief. Some people who used to accept me started to reject me after I got my guide dog. Once Fargo started to come along, people stopped giving me rides. It became harder to attend events, and I would simply stay home.

School was a different matter: I never missed school, even though I would have a three-hour commute both there and back.

Recently I experienced this pain in a religious program I was taking. We were divided into cohorts or small communities of about 10 people. Someone would decide what songs were sung, and another would decide what Scripture passage would be read, and someone else would decide what sermon would be preached. Those who did not have Facebook were left out of the loop—for places to study as a group, or to go to peoples' houses.

The cohort I was in had its little cliques. Some would try to be friendly and they partly succeeded, when I didn't have Fargo. When poor Fargo was part of the mix, people at times would guide me to places if they felt either compelled to do so or, if one of the instructors told them to. When Fargo was there, these seemingly God-fearing, classy, moral adults turned in to childish traitors who sided with each other as to why they couldn't give Fargo and me a ride. They told me that I had to agree with what had happened, and that I should forgive some people, as if nothing had happened!

Things take longer for a blind person—people sometimes forget this, or refuse to even wonder about it.

I felt unwanted in that program. I had angry feelings toward many of the clergy. I wondered why people get such jobs when their life is all about themselves, their job, and their children. I almost doubted God, but I averted those thoughts this time.

I left the program and am now in a better program for me.

No person should feel like they are being shunned.

When a nasty event leaves me feeling ungrounded, I try to rally the forces within me, to cope with the trauma of this type of rejection, the disapproval, and the feeling that no one really has my back anymore since my parents died.

I have strategies. I remind myself that God is good, even though a lot of His people are misguided. I listen to my favourite podcasts and I find ways to enjoy low-budget foods.

I also talk to God and do some fun dialoguing with Fargo. I have a voice for him, when I pet him, and when we talk. I picture him saying comforting things, and I mimic his voice. It cheers me up a lot, and makes the pain easier to bear. I also play guitar if the mood strikes me, or knit, or exercise.

With a guide dog, I know that I will never travel alone. Having guide dogs has taught me to be more curious and empathetic toward people. Having a guide dog tells you who your real friends are.

No matter how much rejection I face, I know I am a good person.

I am fragmented in my faith, and perhaps in my character growth, and perhaps in my views of people, but I realize that there is beauty that shines within me, and shows my redeeming qualities to others, if they are only willing and able to see it.

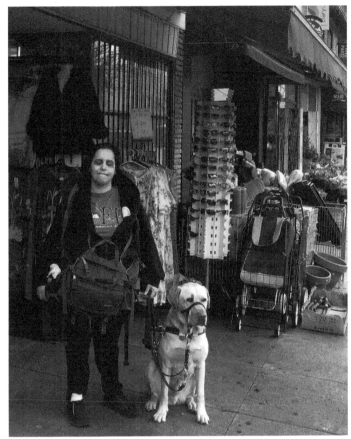

PHOTO BY: PETER O'BRIEN

**Neena Saloya** completed her diploma in Radio Broadcast Technology from Humber College, and an undergraduate degree at the University of Toronto with a major in Christianity in Culture, a minor in Psychology, and a minor in English literature. She has a Masters degree in Theological Studies from Tyndale Seminary. She married Kevin Avery. She recently started a home-based business making soaps, candles, knitted items, beaded jewelry, tactile visual paintings and drawings. Her hobbies include knitting, working out almost every day, reading, listening to podcasts, watching movies with described audio, and listening to music. Her guide dog Fargo is a source of joy, who inspires her to get up and go places daily. She has an eclectic faith, with which she has a love / hate relationship at the best of times.

Ellen

# The
# Miracle of
# Jacob

Schwartz

Do you believe in miracles? I do. Here's why.

Like all young girls, I had dreams and aspirations. When I was really young, I told everyone I wanted to be a famous singer or actress because that seemed like the glamorous choice. Later, I pretended I wanted to be a doctor or lawyer like most of my friends. The truth was that my dream was to be somebody's Mom. I couldn't wait for the day when I could hold and cuddle that newborn child of mine. That day finally arrived when I was 30 years old.

Instead of suffering through a miserable pregnancy, I embraced every single kick and twist from the baby growing inside of me. I loved every minute of those nine months. When my husband Jeff and I met Jacob William Schwartz, our first child, his strapping healthy nine pounds meant that I had arrived, too. My dream had come true.

Like all new parents, we were equally overwhelmed with joy and fear. We went to prenatal classes to help us prepare for anything and everything. For months, I had read articles, books and watched videos about parenthood. There was nothing Jeff and I couldn't handle together. We were a team, and now a healthy threesome, setting out to write the next chapter.

And then, everything changed.

All of the books stated that Jacob's eyes would follow me, the mother. I was the centre of my child's world, the one who bore him, the one who held his milk. His eyes never followed.

All of the books stated that in a few weeks, he would begin to raise his head. We waited and waited. Whenever Jacob tried to lift it, it just flopped back down.

He started crying, and crying, and crying. All of the books stated that colic was a normal part of child development, but the crying didn't stop.

Something was wrong with Jacob.

We were lucky to have a paediatrician who sent us down to the Hospital for Sick Kids in Toronto for a plethora of tests. Jeff and I hugged our two-month-old as doctors and nurses poked and prodded him, hunting for answers.

Why wasn't Jacob meeting the simplest of milestones? What was wrong with Jacob?

Most newborns spend their days cuddled up in a warm blanket in their bassinet or nestled in the loving arms of doting family members. Jacob spent his first months in hospital waiting rooms or lying naked on procedure beds. How could our baby understand what was happening to him when we, his parents, had no idea?

When Jacob was four months old, the hospital called. It was the metabolic and genetics team.

"We have good news and bad news." I asked for the good news first.

"The good news is we know what is wrong with Jacob. The bad news is, it isn't very good news."

Soon, we were sitting in a hospital room, absorbing Jacob's diagnosis and prognosis. "Jacob has a rare, fatal, neurodegenerative illness that attacks the central nervous system. It is called Canavan Disease, a disease for which there is no known treatment or cure. Children with Canavan Disease cannot crawl, walk, sit, or talk. Over time, they may suffer seizures, become paralyzed, or blind, and have trouble swallowing. Death usually occurs before the age of four, although some children may survive into their teens."

In that moment, my dreams for a life of fulfillment and bliss vanished. Hearing the words that our precious boy would never live past the age of four, we braced for a downward spiral. Surely, we were in for a life of sadness, sickness and challenges so huge they'd be too much to handle. Our baby had his whole life ahead and now it felt like a life sentence. Over the years, I have been reminded many times by doctors and therapists, "Remember, Jacob is on borrowed time."

Well, it's a good thing I am terrible at returning things because somehow, some way, the clock ticked on.

Because of Jacob's journey, we have gained lessons about life, about living it in a conscious way, where we have choices about our own actions and perspectives. Somehow, in the depths of life's darkness, a miracle happened.

These lessons did not turn on like a light switch. They came from years of caring for a child with a debilitating illness. The disease robbed Jacob of almost every possible physical and mental ability. The doctors were partially right. Our child couldn't walk, talk, move, or see. He was fed by a tube through his stomach. Because he had a hard time managing his own secretions, his body often needed suctioning. He required one-to-one attention at all times.

When the doctors first delivered the terrible news, we were sure that our lives were over. We were devastated, heartbroken, discouraged. We needed to try something, anything, to help Jacob, and to help ourselves.

There was one chance. We enrolled him in an experimental gene replacement trial at Yale University. It was a risky procedure, but it also gave us a shred of hope. And it turned out to be the "aha" moment we desperately needed in order to go on.

The results were not what we hoped for. Complications from the trial caused Jacob to experience an hour-and-a-half seizure. He spent months lying in a hospital room fighting meningitis and hydrocephalus, his little head wrapped in bandages. Our baby underwent seven operations in two months.

The "aha" moment came after all that. It was when Jeff was lying on his back in the hospital bed with little Jacob stretched out on his daddy's stomach. He was resting inside the safety net of those strong arms wrapped around him, finally sleeping after hours of screaming from the pain. Jeff wouldn't move for fear of waking Jacob, of risking his feeling of peace. It was at that moment when the miracle appeared.

If we could help it, we decided, our child would never experience pain ever again. While we couldn't save Jacob from the disease he was born with, we could accept it and make his life as comfortable and as peaceful as possible. Once we stopped trying to cure Jacob, our lives changed again—this time, for the better. Now, he was the one with the power to help cure us.

It wasn't until I came to grips with that new reality that I realized I had a choice: to accept the life sentence and give up on my dreams or to open up to the possibility of letting new dreams unfold.

Living with someone who has a life-threatening disease is beyond difficult. It can sometimes feel impossible. But in many ways, it is also a gift. It challenges your perspective on life, pushing you to think and act beyond the ordinary.

While I could dwell on the past 21 years of sleepless nights, I choose instead to focus on Jacob's ability to wake up every day. That small blessing, that miracle, drove me to wake up physically, morally, and mentally. And as each day unfolded, Jacob's outlook changed mine. His appreciation for the little things in life helped me to see how miraculous they are. Your attitude in the face of challenge is your choice.

I know that if I am frustrated by misplacing my glasses or car keys, or at my wit's end about the disastrous state of my teenagers' bedrooms or annoyed that Jeff is late for dinner and it's sitting there getting cold, I have a choice. I can let these small upsets brew up inside of me and let them fester into an unnecessary argument that ends up with two sides very unhappy. Or, I can realize that these are just small distractions that truly don't impact anything, other than my nerves. All I had to do is look at Jacob and I was reminded that it had been one amazing day. I try so hard not to dwell on negativity because when I do, the result can only be negative. What good does that do? It only makes the problem worse.

We all have countless choices to make every day—everything from mundane ones such as whether to order dinner or make it from scratch, to bigger ones like whether to leave a secure job to pursue a life-long passion. When it comes to choices, there really are only two options. You can learn from what each life lesson may be teaching you and move forward armed with new knowledge, or pity yourself for your misfortune and move in reverse, missing out on the life lesson altogether.

The hard truth is that life can be tough and unfair, even tragic, but how we get through it is our choice. Whether you are a daughter, son, mother, father, sister or brother, one thing is certain: you will face many unexpected turns, trials and tribulations and it will be how you choose to deal with each one that makes all the difference.

Think of a teeter totter constantly moving up and down, up and down. Imagine if it were balanced all of the time. What fun would that be? The key to life is not in finding balance in everything you do. Instead, it is in finding concrete ways to celebrate and embrace the highs and to learn and grow from the lows. It is in those two extremes that the fun, the growth, and the blessings can be found.

Jacob reveled in every second of every day he was here. He passed away in 2019. Although a large piece of me died that day, his lessons and his love will be with me always. Life with Jacob was a blessing and as long as I am living I will continue to share his messages. He couldn't speak, but we heard him loud and clear. He couldn't see, but he had such vision. He couldn't move, but he was able to move mountains.

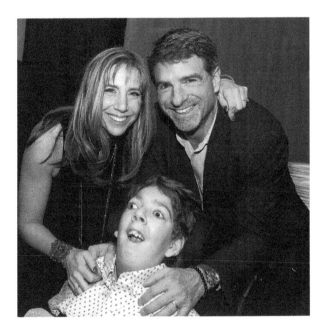

**Ellen Schwartz** is an elementary school teacher and an advocate for individuals with special needs. As founder of Project Give Back she is helping inspire a new generation of empathetic and compassionate young leaders. She is the co-founder of Jacob's Ladder, which has raised over $3 million toward research and education into neurodegenerative illnesses. In 2016 she was awarded a Meritorious Service Decoration by the Governor General of Canada. She wrote *Lessons from Jacob: A Disabled Son Teaches His Mother About Courage, Hope and the Joy of Living Life to the Fullest*, and *Without One Word Spoken*, which became a Canadian best seller on *The Globe and Mail*'s book list.

Kenneth

Four Poems from

# Jogging with the Great Ray Charles

Sherman

HEART

So there you are at last,
on the diagnostician's screen,
fluctuating between clinical grey
and amber, chambers
opening and closing:
a mollusc
kneading its vital fluid.

You look so primitive.
Who would suspect you to inhabit
a human chest, to fasten
with such tenacity
onto memories, lyrics,
frames of an old black
and white film?

Hoarder, I lie awake at night
hearing you *thump thump*
as if you were banging on the door
of my life, pleading
for one more chance
to wipe the slate clean
and begin again.

AWAITING BIOPSY RESULTS

"Suffering," says Simone Weil
"is time without direction."
Light cuts through the blinds
razor-thin. In your state
of suspended animation
you listen for your heart
to beat
for the phone
to ring
for a voice
to call you back
to the living.

## A DREAM OF LEAVING THE TORONTO GENERAL

I arose from my hospital bed
dressed and walked out of my room
and down the corridor

the nurses did not recognize me
how can that be I wondered
I knew I was the colour of a cadaver

In the elevator I stared straight ahead
avoiding the eyes of the orderlies

I walked into the street
and joined the press of people
going their determined ways

It was a comfort to have a direction
my illness had made me desultory,
I had been riding death's wave
and now I was once again like
everyone,
like everyone I strode with the swell
of human traffic
anxious over things
that needed doing

I reached the corner
and fixed eyes with a street singer
I knew no one in life has eyes
that intense that focused
his mouth moved soundless
he strummed silence on his guitar
his plush-lined case

swung open like a coffin
and for a moment I panicked
believing I'd been walking
through the land
of the living dead

I tossed him a coin and kept walking
blending with the crowd
hoping that he could not see
the mark upon me.

VENUS OCCLUDED

I awoke one morning to discover one eye
weird, blurry, as if opened underwater.
At first I thought I was imagining the effect,
denial my reaction to any physical mishap.
But two days later I found myself sitting
in the darkened chamber, the ophthalmologist
hunched over me, his miner's light probing
the flooded landscape of my retina. "There it is."
Then the ominous pause. "A venous occlusion...
some damage..." I understood occlusion as blockage,
but not being from the scientific side of things
or wanting, perhaps, to accept responsibility for failed vision
I heard him speak the name of the Goddess
and wondered if those images were fading
because they'd not been loved enough.

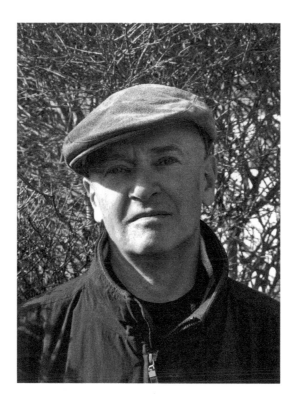

**Kenneth Sherman** is the author of several books of poetry and prose, includ-ing the highly acclaimed long poems, *Words for Elephant Man* and *Black River*. His essay collection, *What the Furies Bring*, won the 2010 Canadian Jewish Book Award. His *Wait Time: A Memoir of Cancer*, was nominated for the 2017 RBC Taylor non-fiction prize. His most recent book is the poetry collection, *Jogging with the Great Ray Charles* (ECW Press). He lives in Toronto where he conducts poetry writ-ing workshops.

charles c.

# waiting
# to explode:
# four poems

smith

*retribution*

how does one arrive again at birth?

you're given a coin for passage
a boat on a quiet summer afternoon

light glancing over the sure lips of water
you float at the wind's will

then watch stars fall into dawn

no one ever tells you who is in control
or that anyone for that matter is

each day is an episode in shadows
nothing in the trees feeds the earth

each crossroad leads to hunger
emptiness in the bowels the spirit leaks

you are covered with such misfortune
you suddenly feel you must
learn from earlier lives

and where they intersect
with the air you now breath

*whispers*

the moon now a faint wisp in the cloud-filled sky
whispers cover the sidewalk and fall into the earth

the green-rusted brass bell tomorrow rings into silence
the dull thud of continuing empire claims so many lives

from evening until night time the same expression
captures the ever-receding tree-lined horizon

the leaves of so many oaks maples birch and willow
litter the expanse and bend into endless fields

what shadows the wild tall grass aspire to contain
those bright lights waiting to explode upon the sleeping hills

*at the edge*

let the wind enter        let the sound at the door
step slowly      into the living room

let your lungs            breath on their own
let your eyes              see what is in and beyond

both cause        and its unknown pedigree -

let the round night        take you thru mist
let its scent       fold into you like a glove -

you will see it then        as anyone might
the difference between   parting the sea to let thru a crowd

and walking on waters   with neither permission nor aid -

alone in one instance                obligation shaping the other
in these spaces   where  legacy gives birth

and crawls like veins            across your biceps
and the back of your hands -

and with what you found there   squeezed dry like paper
you carried yourself            into what could only be

from what was
and will always  and always become

something unmentionable        crumbling about you

at each step        landslides cluttering your way
while everything else            rolls down hills -

*between destinies*

there are times  i wonder what it must have been like
for you  with me inside a full six months and kicking
and him outside  lying flat and still
in a casket  open for two days in a funeral parlour

other times  i think of you spending your night
looking out the bedroom window  into a sky
full of dark promises  and small lights you hoped
he would pass by  so that you could see him
as he would always be  an angel fading into space

and when they lay him  like a boxed parcel
into the gaping  sun-dried earth
you must have felt  torn as no other
between destinies  with a small heart
at work in your womb  and the gentle brown
eyes of a young boy  closed forever

semblances of your pain  must have appeared to you
and i could see you  seeing yourself with
an arm cut off  the blood bursting into a pool
or standing in a field  of fading green
as the earth opened up  below your feet
to suck you in  like a puddle

i was always told  it took six men
to drag you  from that burial
kicking and screaming  how badly you wanted
in  while the earth fell on him like a ton

later you told me  this was something
you would never recover from  and that

your heart beats  like a barking dog
each year  on the day of his death

then you swear  there are moments when
you see him again  thru me
as if he had walked  out of circumstance
into my body  so that when i stand
in front of you  you see a part of him

the earth just could not  swallow

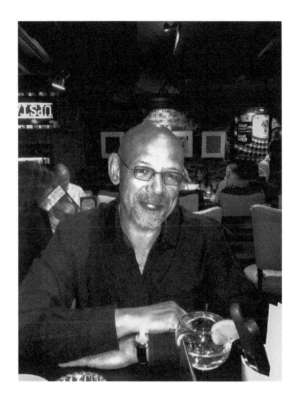

Poet, playwright, and essayist **charles c. smith** has written or edited 14 books. He studied poetry and drama at New York University, and drama at the Frank Silvera's Writers' Workshop in Harlem. charles was the founder of the Black Perspectives Cultural Program in Regent Park, Toronto. His research has been commissioned by the African Canadian Community Coalition on Racial Profiling, the Court Challenges Program of Canada, and the Ontario Ministries of the Attorney General and Community Safety. charles is currently the Executive Director for Cultural Pluralism in the Arts Movement Ontario and Artistic Director of the *wind in the leaves collective*. His book, *Pluralism in the Arts in Canada: A Change is Gonna Come*, was released in June 2012. His book of poetry, *travelogue of the bereaved*, was published in 2014, and his latest non-fiction book *The Dirty War: The Making of the Myth of Black Dangerousness* was released in 2014 by the Canadian Centre for Policy Alternatives.

Rabbi Yael

# Sermon for
# the Second Day of
# Rosh Hashanah
# 2015 / 5776

Splansky

Some might think the best pretext for this sermon is the following Yiddish proverb: "If God lived on earth, people would break His windows." But I prefer another Yiddish proverb instead: "If things are not as you wish, wish them as they are." When I stood before you last Rosh Hashanah it was a great celebration of pride and purpose, of how far we had come as a congregation. We were just beginning to write a new chapter in the life of Holy Blossom Temple. The dominant emotions for me then were excitement and gratitude and curiosity. In the quiet moments of personal reflection then, I privately admitted to myself that seeing our congregation through transition was the hardest thing I had ever done. In my private prayers last Rosh Hashanah I thanked God for giving me the strength to endure it and for the many good partners along the way. Today, one year later, on this Rosh Hashanah, in the quiet moments of personal reflection over another year gone, I can say that now, fighting cancer is the hardest thing I have ever done. God willing, 5776 will be simpler.

I could use a little less excitement, but as the Yiddish proverb goes: "Even the smoothest path is full of stones." No life is free from pain. Even hard-working and kind-hearted rabbis are not protected from *tzuros*. I've never spoken of it from this *bimah* in these many months. Those who know me know that I am a pretty private person. A rabbi's primary purpose is, of course, to teach text. Today, however, the text I bring to share with you is the text of my life. For nine months now, biology and chemistry have been my Torah. Our sages say one cannot fully understand Torah unless one has stumbled in it. Many people encourage me with compliments and say: "How graceful!" but the path has been rocky. There have been many moments when I felt myself stumbling in the Torah of life's hard knocks. But I did not fall.

Before I continue, not another word until I acknowledge that among us are many dear congregants who have truly suffered and are carrying much heavier burdens, and for a lot longer than I have. I look at you, and I see real pillars of strength. Who among us has not accompanied a loved one along one rough road or another, or another? My story, by contrast, is not unique. Unfortunately, it is very common. And in my heart of hearts I believe that my story will have a happy ending. I pray that through these few reflections you may find something familiar and affirming, or something challenging and motivating, or perhaps, the simple comfort in knowing that we are indeed, all in it together. Each one, doing our best to muscle our way through this God-given life.

In preparing for today, I found this in my computer. I had forgotten that I had written it. 4:53 am March 12, 2015: *I like to see all the shades of gray, and consider them. I like to weigh them out against one another. That's how I've always been and as a rabbi, that's my training. My life now, however, is a strange exercise in juxtapositions. A collision of extremes. I am, on the one hand, utterly shocked and disbelieved by my diagnosis, and at the same time, I am not at all surprised. "Hello cancer, I've been expecting you. Not so soon, but expecting you none the less. Why not me?"*

*I feel on the one hand, lucky and also unlucky. I am prepared and I am woefully unprepared. I feel confident that all will go well for me, and I feel totally vulnerable. I am surrounded by so much support: family, congregation, old friends and new, colleagues, strangers, medical experts of all kinds, and on the other hand, sometimes I am entirely alone. At the end of the day, I am the only one in my skin. On the one hand, I hate the machines and the tests and the new books on my shelf, and the needles, and the hospitals and the medicines, and on the other hand, I love them. I am so grateful for them. On the one hand, I feel strong, sometimes even triumphant, on top of it, and there are days when I feel myself pinned down under the weight of it, crushed with worry. I don't want any part of this . . . none of it. But I don't get to choose. A friend who knows, calls it a "choice-less choice."*

Now I don't keep a journal . . . this is really the only thing like this in my computer. Many have advised me to keep a journal. They say you grow, and it's a journey. They say cancer changes you. They say you come out on the other side stronger and wiser. Truth be told, I thought I was already pretty strong and wise. And that's primarily because I have learned from you, good people. Throughout our 17 years together, studying Torah together, inviting me into your lives at delicate moments of trouble and trial, you have taught me well, about vulnerability and vitality. You have trusted me with your insights of fear and faith, and I am stronger and wiser because of you, my teachers.

So today, I try to reciprocate in one small measure, something of what I have learned. This experience reinforces what I already knew to be true. When a congregant wrote to me about her own illness this year, and confessed that she felt paralysed by the deepest, darkest fear that she was somehow being punished by God, I wrote the following:

> Dear Laura, (today I'll call her Laura) I am so sorry to hear about what you are facing. I'm glad that you trust me with your big questions. Email is a lousy way to talk about such important and nuanced things. I look forward to the day when we can sit together and really talk. But in the meantime, since I hear the urgency in your voice, let me say that I do not believe illness is punishment. (Full stop.) I believe that you are a very good person. But even if you were a miserable human being, I do not believe illness would come your way as a result. I believe that illness is as much a part of life as is good health. And I don't mind sharing with you that I write you at a time when I'm facing my own frightening diagnosis.
>
> The question is not, why do bad things happen to good people. The question is, <u>when</u> bad things happen to good people, how do we respond? We don't get to choose when or where cancer cells grow, but we do get to choose how to respond when they do. Do we choose to be proactive or passive? Private or public? Optimistic or pessimistic? Fearful or courageous? These are very personal decisions. Some moments this way, some moments that way. Even when there is so much outside of our control, some things we must remember, are within our control. Some things we can choose. I know that you are blessed with family and friends, and a community that cares about you very much. While you're the only one who lives in your own skin, you are not alone. One of my many prayers for you, Laura, is that you will feel less alone and less frightened. Would you take comfort in knowing that we are including your name in our *Mi Shebeirach* this Shabbat? Yes, of

course, I will keep you in my own private prayers. I ask that you do the same for me. That's the power of sacred community. That's another thing I believe in wholeheartedly.

Be well, Laura. *Refuah Shleimah*. A complete and whole healing. Yael.

This exchange between two moms came about because in a synagogue community we are not alone. This is the essential blessing of being a part of such a community. I always knew this to be true, but this year I experienced it in new ways, as a mother and a wife. I know my husband and our boys are less afraid and more supported because they are a part of this congregation, not because they are the rabbi's kids, but because they're around, and people know them and care about them. Just one example comes in the form of meals that the *Bikur Cholim* Committee arranges for us. Nutritious and delicious meals, prepared by generous congregants and dropped at the door from time to time. These have saved Adam and me some precious time and energy when we needed to conserve. But more than the practical benefits, each meal was a lesson to us and to our children in the power of sacred community. Without family in town, we were buoyed by the embrace of the Holy Blossom congregation. This quiet mitzvah speaks volumes about the character of our congregation.

Now I will never know why cancer settled in my body. I will do everything I can to keep it from returning. But God only knows. So, my faith fills in the gap between the known and the unknown. Between the facts of life and the mysteries of life. There's a blessing for this: *Baruch Atah Adonai, Chacham HaRazim*. Praised are You, Adonai, our God, Ruler of the Universe, Knower of Secrets. To say this *b'rachah* is somehow liberating. I don't have to know everything, because God does.

Since my earliest childhood memories, I have always experienced prayer as something very real. Not foolish, not an empty ritual, not a crutch, but very powerful. But I have never been the subject of people's prayers until now. I have to say, to my surprise, that the accumulation of these prayers somehow have substance. They have volume and weight and largesse. It's difficult for me to articulate, actually. They add up to something almost tangible, for me. So I want to thank you this day for holding me in your prayers. They have indeed sustained me. And I want to suggest, that if you have loved ones who are unwell, instead of saying to them, "I am thinking about you all the time," let them know that you are praying for them all the time. Thinking about is a form of praying about. And you'd be surprised how much it will mean to them.

I personally don't pray for God to rescue me. I pray for God to make me strong. Never before was my experience of God bodily, as it has been this year. I never said like Job, "Through my flesh I see God." Until my diagnosis, my encounters with the Divine were through my head and my heart and my *neshamah*, but now my hair and my fingernails and my white blood cells and lymph nodes I never knew I had, all have something to report to me. Every miraculous thing, every quirky side effect, every achy joint points to the wonder and the mystery of God's world and the God-given ability to heal.

One congregant among you brought me a gift from Israel. A thin, little red bracelet, with a Hamsa on it. Now I am not a superstitious person. I do not believe that the red thread will ward off the evil eye. I do not believe the little silver hand will protect or shield me from harm. But I've been wearing this little gift every day, nonetheless. I'll tell you why I wear it. It's a reminder to me that I must do all that I can to protect myself from harm. Remember to eat, remember to drink, remember to sleep. The little blue eye at the centre of the Hamsa stands for God's watchful eye. I see it, I look upon it, and I hear the voice in the back of my mind saying, "Are you taking care, Yael? Your family and congregation need you for the long haul, you know." And usually that's enough to get me on the treadmill. That is prayer in motion.

Another Yiddish proverb: "Chutzpah succeeds." With my doctor's permission, I have pushed myself to work as much as I could throughout chemo. I take one week off and then have two weeks back at work, and that pattern continues for each cycle. So far I've been lucky with daily radiation. In fact, I have my afternoon appointment calling me soon. It feels good to work. It feels good to do for, to apply myself to something other than myself, to give myself to others, not only to give to myself. It is good to be reminded of who I am, not only as a patient. My work is a reminder that I am alive.

Moments ago, we read from the High Holy Day Prayerbook, *Adam Yissodo*, "You have created us and You know what we are but flesh and blood. Man's origin is dust and dust is his end. Each of us is a shattered urn, grass that must wither, a flower that will fade, a shadow moving on, a cloud passing by, a particle of dust floating on the wind, a dream soon forgotten."

*V'atah Hu Melech El Chai v'Kayam.* "But You, O God, are the Sovereign One, the Everlasting God." This beautiful and haunting prayer-poem contrasts our fleeting days to God's eternality. And it is not a fatalist's prayer. Make no mistake . . . just the opposite. It says that we have a chance at eternity. By attaching ourselves to the Eternal God, when we create for ourselves, day in and day out, (as hard as it is) a life of meaning and purpose, we can cross the divide from suffering to service. That is every person's sacred task.

The composers and compilers of our *Machzor* did not intend to traumatize us, so don't mistake my tears today. They only wanted to speak the truth as they knew it, so that we might live more fully. We might read that prayer poem and ask, "Okay, so I'm mortal. Nu?" And the *Machzor* says back to us, "So what are you going to do about it?" Yes, we are only dust, but dust can make for a strong foundation on which we can build a house, or even a synagogue. We may be broken vessels, but those shards can be reassembled and reconfigured to create a beautiful mosaic. And yes, we are withering grass and wilting flowers, but these enrich the soil that is beneath so that life can renew and emerge. And yes, we are but a shadow. The Psalmist says "Our days on earth are like a shadow." And one commentator asks, "So what kind of shadow is that?" And the answer comes, "Not a shadow cast by a wall, not a shadow cast by a tree, but as a shadow cast by a bird flying overhead." Let the shadow that we are be a sign of life, and of movement and mission. *Adam Yissodo* is placed in out *Machzor* between prayers devoted to the themes of *G'vurot* and *K'dushah* . . . courage and holiness. That is right where the sick and those who love them reside, wedged right in between courage and holiness.

Each Shabbat, we end our services with the words of *Adon Olam*. "Into Your hands, O God, I entrust my spirit, and when I sleep and when I wake, and with my spirit and my body too, as long as God is with me, I shall not

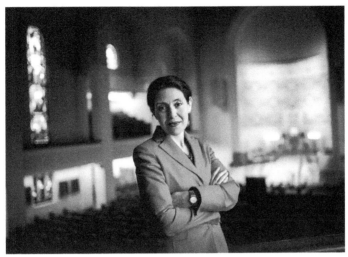

PHOTO BY: MARK BLINICH

fear." For the mountains may crumble and the hills may shake, but my love will never leave you, God says. Things fall apart, but God's presence is steady, and faithful.

O God of life, we pray that You will write us into the Book of Life, so that we may live. Strengthen our bodies and our souls so that we are able to fill our days in Your service. And that we might make every day a *Shechehianu.*

Together: *Baruch, Atah Adonai, Elohenu Melech Ha Olam Shehechiyanu v'kiyemanu v'higiyanu, lazman hazeh.* Praised are you Adonai, Our God, Ruler of the Universe, who has given us this good life, who sustains us each day, and who has enabled us to reach this moment so filled with joy and blessing. Amen.

———

**Yael Splansky** is the Senior Rabbi of Holy Blossom Temple in Toronto. She is the editor of the prayer book, *Siddur Pirchei Kodesh,* and is a regular contributor to *The Canadian Jewish News.* She is a fourth generation Reform Rabbi. Together with her husband Adam Sol, she raises three sons.

Michelle

# A Song
# Dreams
# Within

Sylliboy

A song dreams within a story
along each web of circumstance
we make our way through a weave
as if a sentient being challenged us centuries ago
of nightly whispers
to fly over mountains
as they watch from afar
a balancing act
awaiting your arrival to the other side

When the time came to tell the story of survival, my body self was tired of understanding the challenges that shaped my existence, as if trauma no longer mattered. Undetermined and as far away as the next galaxy. Trauma to my adult self could only be described as an inheritance from birth, blood memories that flow in and out of the pending doom towards the inevitable. You cry over nothing, burst into a badly sung song because you neglected your vocal chords, being homeless during the tumultuous teen years.

My heart is a riddle waiting to be solved
sing me songs to freedom
carry me across your threshold to love and sanity
creatively introducing me to excel by prospering
truth-telling energies exchanging secrets of our past
will we meet when we are ready
half a century is knocking on my door soon
Trauma took away my ability to love
Trauma took away my ability
to be healthy with another person
Trauma paid its respects to our dearly beloved
Trauma tricked me not to exist for a long time

When you are born a First Nations person, you lose track of the number of funerals you attend. Funeral pressures towards grief never last for too long. Picture your spiritual being taking your pressures away to another existence. I'm not afraid of death when it's time to leave this world—that is what nature intended. There is an old memory of meeting someone at a funeral for the first time, someone who affected my heart in a big way. That was the day my heart was ripped wide open to what we call feelings. Strange place to experience feelings at a funeral. Vulnerability already existed, so it was easy. When you are born from a woman who experienced trauma because of residential school. You are born with her memories, and you are left to wonder if the memories you are experiencing are yours or hers, especially when pain and suffering come out of nowhere and with no explanation.

There is a tragic influence that vibrates from within when there is no emotion to the event that took someone's life so suddenly. As a child, many years ago, a foster kid in my grandfather's home took away my innocence after years of healing. I'm no longer a daily victim of the unwanted event. Perhaps the reason is existential: he died years later. Unfortunately other abusers came and went, but he was the first to influence my upbringing. The forced changes endured as a child and as a youth were traumatic, critical and unnecessary. No one in my family knew of the abuse—no one accept me and my step-sister, who was there when it happened. We carried our secret to her grave. To this day I don't remember why we never told adults. He must've threatened us. Who knows, my memories are scarce.

How does one heal as a child in a reservation filled with many worlds of possibilities? My saving grace was not the support of therapy or counselling, it was reading novels. The book mobile that came to my community was my first escape, the second was me running away. Every novel reminded me that creativity gave you permission to escape, simply by reading someone else's adventures. A cleverly disguised gift that allowed me an ability to create something out of nothing years later as an artist. To live in the imaginary allows you to heal.

Step into a world
that place of wonder where
we are always dreaming
perhaps my safety

is to dream daily
allowing my spirit
to be adventurous

An instant passed just now, a sign that resembles monotone colours of existence creating a moment of gratitude, an ability to express freely without a care in the world. My mind is wandering, snow is gently falling from the sky covering my beautiful west coast city.

Having faith in spirit and the ancestors is easy for me to acknowledge, speaking with them daily is part of my ritual. There are no qualms about the reasons that exist between worlds. The silence and the meditation is part of my answer to every logical explanation, because in my world it habitually exists. A skeptic would say trauma gave you that reasoning, you only believe because you were traumatized as a child. Knowledge dictates a certain way for everyone on this planet. Indigenous pedagogy is not sensory, but an advocate to spirit the right to express without prejudice. Dawn arrives as easily as the sunsets. Whatever happens in-between is up to you as an individual. You are never alone.

Spirit speaks
Spirit visits
Spirit acknowledges

As a young adult the gifts inherited from my biological mother emerged with full force. The path was laid out to be the go-between among spirit and existence. For a short time my job was to help those who did not realize they had moved on to the spirit realm. The task was not simple. It was powered with huge responsibility. When the gift became overwhelming, my inexperienced young self had to tell my ancestors. The job they assigned to me was too much for a young person with no guide or teacher. Once the declaration for it to stop was made, the spirits stopped coming, my duties complete. For many years, when memories emerged of my decision to stop, I wondered what my life would have been like had a teacher not been available to guide me with my gifts.

The art of freedom
is gaining inner peace
a patchwork of solitude
of how the world spins
despite our pleas for hope
sacrifice from an undemanding spiritual realm
universal code of love and harmony
clears a pathway when asked
by summoning the gods of within
they too understand our voices
of how blood flows
an ultimate journey
we are meant to complete

Healing, from residential school effects, does not happen overnight. It took elders revealing their stories to help me understand how it affected my life as a child. The stories told in public were not mine, but they affected me in ways only a person who is a child of a residential school survivor would understand. The challenge for me was to understand my own family, people and history. When you are part of history. The first step towards healing is recognizing the connection, that you are an intergenerational survivor coming to grips with the trauma of what your parents endured, and not your own. These confusing revelations are stories yet to be told. The stories Canadians heard about elder experiences at residential school were not about the intergenerational effects, they were stories about their experiences. My mother's mental health prevented me and my siblings in knowing what really happened to her in residential school. Her inability to cope was proof that she never needed to tell her story to anyone ever again.

If the stories from total strangers is all you have to go on, how does one heal when reconciliation is a constant theme in everyone's vocabulary? Who am I healing for: myself or my departed mother? Reconciliation involves two sides. What happens when you cannot confront the other side?

Seventy thousand people marched across the bridge for reconciliation, after the Truth and Reconciliation Conference in Vancouver. The only strength left in me after my family got on the plane was to sit on a bench on Commercial Drive and cry. What happened on that bench allowed healing fingers to tap until the tears stopped.

Fall equinox spoke to me today
September 22, 2013

It will die, my phone will die
(100% remains)
yet it will die,
good news is, it will be resurrected an hour later
by hydro-electric power grids that drowned mother earth centuries ago

water was not born to destroy
(99% remains)

sacred calls: why are you different
questions need answers, my answers will die
(98% remains)

mother speaks, child listens
mother died
(97% remains)

don't you get it, oil destroys, one day it too will die
(96% remains)

father died, child had no answers
(95% remains)

sons of daughters played with their own memories
(94% remains)

lifecycle, tell me a story,
why is my mind having a hard time letting go
(90% remains)

do we shout without meaning sacrifice, heart, sacrifice
(87% remains)

underneath the stairwell policy notes are left behind
(85% remains)

visiting other worlds has meaning
(80% remains)

anger hovers above rain clouds reminding me to cleanse
(79% remains)

talk to me again, ancestors, your visits are welcomed anytime
(75% remains)

ambivalent discombobulated
(70% remains)

we cry when energies are too much for the soul
(69% remains)

feeling altruistic, uncommon values exist
(65% remains)

trauma lays dormant for years like an unwelcomed visitor
(62% remains)

soldier laid down gun, is suddenly accused of treason,
refusing to kill on behalf of half-truths and corporate greed
(60% remains)

we die a little each day only to be reborn the next
(57% remains)

tears are comforting, go ahead, ask me how I am doing
(55% remains)

comfort me sweetness only
(50% remains)

confiscating values for profit
(49% remains)

diluted river is driven to madness
(45% remains)

inconsistency is not acceptable
(40% remains)

failure was not an option
my heart only wanted love
(39% remains)

understanding healing as a means to an end
(35% remains)

talking to an elder about how I really feel today
(30% remains)

uncontrolled madness takes a stab at decency,
retroactive to the day she was born
(27% remains)

do they hear what is really going on inside my head
(25% remains)

pain is stored for process,
like an undeveloped hypothesis waiting to emerge
(22% remains)

lines are crossed, purpose unraveled
(19% remains)

running away was not my first option
(15% remains)

staring at darkness only to be brought back alive
by wires that make no sense
(10% remains)

reaching out to love on a day that made no sense
(5% remains)

having the ability to feel
(1% remains)

removing barriers, allowing room to breathe peace
(0% remains)

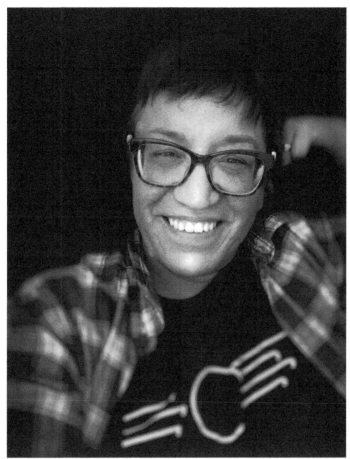

PHOTO BY: KAROLINA TUREK

Interdisciplinary artist and poet **Michelle Sylliboy** (Mi'kmaq/L'nu) was born in Boston, Massachusetts, and raised on her traditional L'nuk territory in We'koqmaq, Cape Breton. While living on the traditional, unceded territories of the Musqueam, Squamish, and Tsleil-Waututh Nations, Sylliboy completed a BFA at Emily Carr University of Art + Design, and a Master's in Education from Simon Fraser University. She is currently a PhD candidate in Simon Fraser University's Philosophy of Education program, where she is working to reclaim her original written komqwej'wikasikl language. Her collection of photography and Mi'kmaq (L'nuk) hieroglyphic poetry, *Kiskajeyi—I Am Ready*, was published by Rebel Mountain Press in 2019.

Andrea

# Honouring Aunt Catherine, and Beyond

Warnick

The course of my life was irrevocably changed on a February day in 1988 when I learned that my Aunt Catherine had died from cancer.

I had known her death was coming. The year earlier, at age 10, I'd had a conversation with my dad, her older brother. I knew about Terry Fox and I asked my dad: "Will Aunt Catherine die of her cancer?" He said: "Yes, she will."

Knowing someone will die doesn't eliminate the surprise, the disbelief, when it actually happens. Catherine's death knocked my world off balance. I barricaded myself into the bathroom and wailed. I was flooded with feelings that I had never encountered before. There was sorrow and anger, and other feelings I didn't have a name for. A sense of how powerless we are in the face of mortality.

Catherine's death was my first real introduction to how unfair the world could be, and to how the most important things in life don't follow the effort-reward model. At the time, my overwhelming feelings of devastation and injustice were because my cousins, Joanna aged 5 and Paula aged 10, had just experienced the death of their mom.

Like most children, I was a sponge for all that was going on around me: the conversations about how to support my cousins, the well-intentioned attempts by the adults in the days following her death to "keep them busy having fun so they don't have time to be sad," and the decision to not have them attend her funeral. My cousins and I lived across the country from one another, and Paula and I wrote letters to keep in touch between visits. When I asked about how to best acknowledge her mother's death in my first letter to Paula after Catherine died, my dad gently advised me not to mention their mom at all. He was concerned that it would cause them to feel sad. This advice didn't sit well with me, but I was too young to understand the source of my discomfort, let alone articulate it. I followed his advice, unaware that the stage had just been set in our family for years of Catherine's death being a topic that no one talked about.

My dad Bill was a wonderful man with a huge heart and a love of adventure. His sense of loyalty for his family, including his extended family, ran deep, and there was little he wouldn't do for his nieces and nephews. He was 46 when his sister died. While at Catherine's funeral, he concluded that life was too short to live far away from both his sister's family and the mountains and the ocean that had been calling him for years. After the funeral, my parents announced that our family of four (plus one geriatric cat) was moving across the country, from Toronto to Vancouver, where we would live just minutes away from Paula, Joanna, and their dad, Neil.

Although Catherine's death was not a topic of discussion in our family, it was frequently on my mind. I wanted to hear her name, and I wondered if others were thinking about her death as much as I was. I wanted to talk about her, her death, and how it impacted everyone, especially her husband and kids. Yet I followed the lead of the adults around me, and rarely brought her up.

I wondered if our efforts to protect Paula and Joanna from the sadness of their mom's death were misguided. They hadn't been told that their mom had cancer, or that she was dying. Catherine's approach was likely rooted in her desire to protect her kids as long as possible from the reality of her impending death. I struggled with feeling disloyal to Catherine by even internally questioning her approach of keeping this devastating reality from her children, yet a deep curiosity was brewing in me as how best to support kids who experience the death of a parent. I turned to literature to explore the topic, and before I was even a teen I started to read anything I could get my hands on about cancer, dying, and grief support for kids.

I continued to read such books throughout my teenaged years, including *On Children and Death* (Elisabeth Kübler-Ross), *The Death of Ivan Illyich* (Leo Tolstoy), and *The Private World of Dying Children* (Myra Bluebond-Langner). These and related books opened my eyes to our society's strong tendency towards denying death, and the sense of isolation that can result both for the person who is dying and those who are closest to that person. Some books also shed light on what happens when children are relegated to the sidelines and denied access to information about the illness or death. Without access to accurate information in an age-appropriate manner, children use their imaginations to help them understand what is happening in their family. These explanations can be wildly inaccurate, causing even more distress.

One of the stories I read during this time was a *Reader's Digest* non-fiction story written by a mother about her young daughter who died of cancer, and the nurse who took care of her at the end of her life. Something stirred in me, and as I read this story I decided that I wanted to be a paediatric oncology nurse. I envisioned myself at the hospital bedside of kids with cancer, supporting them through the illness, and in some cases, their own death.

Ten years later I was doing just that. I spent my twenties working in various cities and countries as a nurse in both paediatric and adult oncology. It didn't take me long to gain insight into the fact that my aunt and uncle likely didn't receive any information at all on how to support their children through Catherine's five years of living with cancer. In the worlds of adult and paediatric oncology there was little emphasis on how to communicate information about the diagnosis and prognosis to children. The focus was predominantly on "conquering cancer," or the science of medicine, with little room left over for the art of medicine. The language being employed in the hospital wards could easily give one the impression of being in a warzone. Words such as "fight," "battle," and "conquer" were spoken by staff and families, despite the unintended implication that dying from the disease involved "giving up" or "not fighting hard enough."

When all treatment options were exhausted, I observed a sense of an impending death representing a medical failure for the health care team. A heartbreaking one, and one that brought compassion from the team, but for many health care providers that compassion was accompanied by significant discomfort. Discomfort about what to say to the family, how to bear witness to their emotional devastation, and an uncertainty about how to best support the family and child through the dying process. Even when death was staring us in the face, use of the "d" word was avoided by nurses, physicians, and social workers alike. The fact that Bluebond-Lagner identified back in the '70s that children as young as three who have leukemia tend to know when they are dying, was a piece of academic knowledge that hadn't translated to any change in practice on the paediatric oncology wards. Bluebond-Lagner's observations shed light on the tendency that young children have an awareness of their dying, and that they also try to conceal this awareness from parents and medical staff. She also observed how adults try to conceal their awareness of their child's impeding death. I witnessed this charade play out with many of the families who I worked with.

Catherine's story was ever-present in my mind. It became increasingly clear to me that I wanted my life work to focus on improving the support families received, particularly within the health care system, both prior to and following a death.

One day I found myself in an internet café in a town on the eastern coast of Tanzania, looking up "master's degrees in dying and death." Within seconds I was introduced to the word "thanatology": the study of dying and death. I was immediately intrigued, and within a year was living in Maryland pursuing the degree, despite having no idea as to where having a "master's in death" would lead.

A decade has now passed since I completed my master's degree in Thanatology, a discipline that is often called the "scientific study of death," but in my experience is far more steeped in the arts: sociology, psychology, anthropology. Through a combination of luck, experience, and passion I've been able to build a career that involves counselling families grieving an illness or death, and providing education to institutions, organizations, and communities. There is no shortage of work to be done. The gap between theory and practice remains significant. Even today far too few families receive well-informed guidance on how to best support children when there is an illness or death in the family.

I am, however, beginning to sense a shift occurring in the public consciousness which is slowly dismantling the attitude of death-denial that is so prevalent in Western society. Conversations about dying and death are increasingly becoming a part of the public discourse, from "medical assistance in dying" to "death cafés," to "advanced care planning" and "home funerals." There is an increasing recognition of children's wisdom and willingness, when adults meet them with warmth and honesty, to engage in discussions about dying and death, and to openly wonder about one of life's biggest mysteries: our morality. Though not always translated into practice, the rights of children and youth to have access to information about their own health and the health of their family members is becoming more recognized, and in some countries even translated into legislation. Researchers are increasingly engaging youth directly to explore their experiences of grief when a family member is ill, dying, or has died. The message of the youth is clear: they benefit from preparation, honesty, and inclusion.

In my practice, children as young as three years old express a desire to know not only the name of a loved one's illness, but how the illness works, and what to expect as the person gets closer to dying. Many of these children have shared with me their explanations for the illness in their family such as "My mom yelled at me so much to clean up my room, that it caused her to get throat cancer" or "I stressed my dad out and he got ALS." These kids are visibly relieved to learn that not only did they not cause the illness, they also can't catch it from the person.

Some kids want to be at the bedside of a dying sibling or parent even at the time of death, and some want time alone with the person's body after death. But most children won't take the lead in asking for these ways of being involved: an adult needs to open up the conversation and offer such options.

Most of the children in my practice benefit from attending a loved one's funeral or memorial, and also participating in it, either by speaking at the ceremony or putting something into the casket: a note, drawing, photo, or some other object of importance.

Supporting grieving children and families entails finding a delicate balance between bearing witness to their emotional pain (as opposed to trying to fix it) and offering well-informed guidance aimed at helping children understand the illness, dying and death, feel included in all that is unfolding, and remain connected to the person who died. When this balance is accomplished, children's stories can be shaped in a way that promotes resilience and an ability to still thrive in life.

Catherine likely never received any such guidance on how to best support her kids during her five years of having cancer. While I am hopeful that we are moving closer to a time in which it will be standard practice to offer parents evidence-based information on how to best support their children when there is a serious illness or death in the family, I am also aware that there is still much work to be done in order to bridge the current knowledge and practice gap. Engaging in such life work, which also allows me to enter people's lives at such a significant and intimate time, is something I feel deeply privileged to do. Every day, when I connect with families and health care professionals to offer support and information that aims to engage and acknowledge children's needs, I am, in my own way, paying tribute to my Aunt Catherine and my own family's experience.

In a sense, I remain that 11-year-old girl wondering about death.

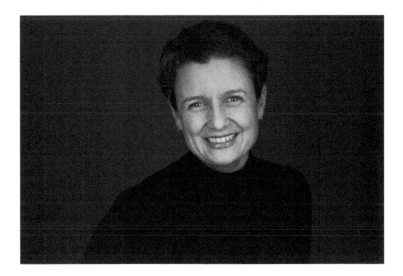

**Andrea Warnick** is an educator and grief therapist who is passionate about ensuring that people of all ages have access to caring and informed support when experiencing the dying or death of someone close to them. As a registered psychotherapist with a degree in nursing and a master's degree in Thanatology, Andrea brings to her work a rare mixture of medical and psychosocial expertise. Andrea runs her own business, Andrea Warnick Consulting and lives in Southern Ontario with her partner and daughters. When not talking about issues related to dying and death she can be found raising monarch caterpillars in an ongoing quest to increase the monarch butterfly population.

Paul

# Children

Watson

I was investigating persistent reports in the disputed territory of Kashmir of men disappearing at the hands of Indian security forces when I met Madan Lal, 65, in Mangu Chak on November 9, 2005. Sitting in the dusty yard of his small home, Lal began to sob as he told me of the anonymous informant who claimed his son Bushan, 25, was murdered along with three other Hindu porters in an alleged "false encounter" with separatist insurgents, which human rights workers said were staged often to boost the body count. Lal was coming to terms with his son's unexplained death. What tore at his heart now was the mystery of how he would care for the dead man's two young daughters. One sitting next to him locked onto me with fierce eyes, burning with such intense fear and anger, that she sent a chill through me. Fear, anger and deep distrust were infecting a new generation, poisoning any hope for peace.

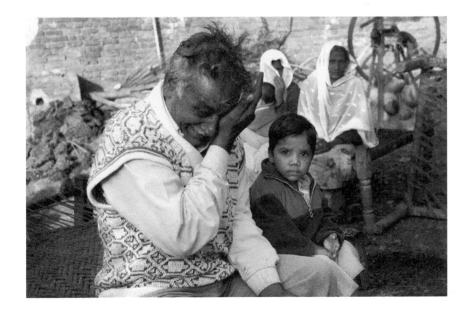

A magnitude-7.6 earthquake viciously shook northern Pakistan on October 8, 2005, killing more than 80,000 people and leaving another 2.5 million without homes. Four days after the quake struck, when the dazed and wounded were still emerging from the rubble on October 12, 2005, I watched as doctors in Dherkot cleaned and sewed up the deep gash that a falling rock slashed across 8-year-old Keala Khan's forehead. For just a moment, his screams stopped and he warily focused on my lens, as if he now feared I was the next to hurt him. Then he shivered with another searing jolt of pain and his screams echoed again through the poorly equipped mountain clinic. In a way, Keala was fortunate. Weeks later, on December 16, 2005, I reached the remote mountain village of Bandi Peza, where families were struggling to survive freezing winter weather. Shivering children had no winter coats, gloves or even socks to warm exposed feet in cracked plastic shoes.

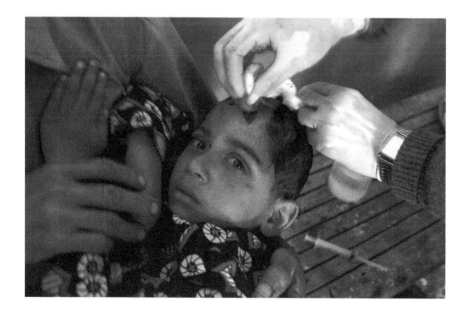

Just over two weeks after a magnitude-7.6 earthquake devastated northern Pakistan, I came across Mohammed Wali, 53, walking along the roadside in the Jhelum River valley that flows through Pakistan-controlled Kashmir. He held his 2-year-old daughter Zakia Bibi tightly to his chest. Wali had hiked seven hours down a mountain trail in a frantic trek for medical care on October 23, 2005. At first, looking only in the little girl's eyes, I saw serenity, not fear. But then she turned her head, and I winced at the gaping wound that a hunk of collapsing concrete had sliced deep into her soft cheek. My mind raced back to Rwanda where, 11 years earlier, I had photographed countless corpses of children with similar wounds, hacked by the machete blades of genocidal murderers. Zakia's pain must have been excruciating. I'm sure it was shock that quieted her. Yet she was also strong in silence, her eyes bright, without a single tear to streak the dirt that covered her beautiful face. The terror was in her father's eyes. He knew his little girl needed help fast to beat an infection that could quickly kill her.

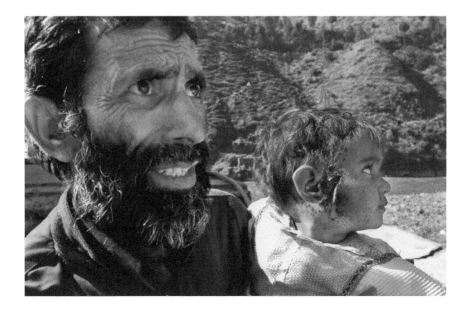

During the U.S.-led invasion to remove Iraqi President Sadaam Hussein's regime in 2003, I entered from Iran into the predominantly Kurdish north to follow the advance of Peshmerga fighters supported by units of American Special Forces. The day after the capital Baghdad fell far to the south, the allied forces took control of Kirkuk in the north on April 10, 2003. Sadaam's troops didn't put up much of a fight, but there was a lot of bloodshed anyway. While U.S. Special Forces focused on securing 300 oil wells outside the city, to prevent the toppling regime from setting them ablaze, loyalist soldiers and Kurdish fighters clashed in the city's streets. Caught in the crossfire were innocents like the dying girl I found in the city's main hospital, overflowing with wounded and the dead. A girl in an orange dress lay on a blood-stained bed with a severe head wound wrapped in gauze. A doctor lifted a closed eyelid with his thumb and I could see the child's life slipping away. "I would like to fly in the sky. I'm so happy," Ali Hussin Ali, told me in a crowded street nearby. "Today, we have freedom." By late afternoon, the hospital had taken in at least 50 gunshot victims. An ambulance driver told me they were all civilians. At least some—maybe even the dying girl— were struck by bullets that fell like rain from the sky in celebratory gunfire.

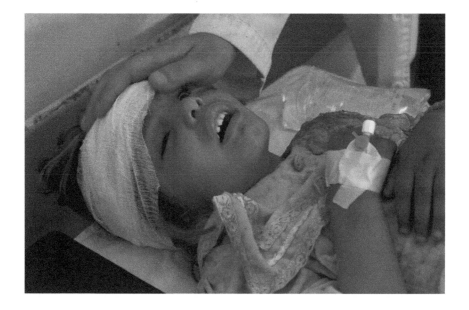

Some of Myanmar's poorest people live by the rivers in northern Kachin state where panning for flakes of gold is the only way to make money for many villagers. I had to sneak into the country as a tourist, and travel undercover, because the military regime didn't want the outside world to know the truth of places like Myit-Son, where the Mali and N'Mai Rivers, fed by Himalayan glaciers, converge in remote northern Burma. The generals and their families were getting very rich off exports of jade, rubies and sapphires. The poor people of Myit-Son were left with the scraps. On December 10, 2007, I watched children who squatted for long hours each day by the riverside, panning for gold in the swirling eddies, instead of going to school to learn to read and write. One child, still too young to work, but facing the same future in a few short years, padded toward me in bunny ears. Her face and yellow dress smeared with the soil of a cruel life, she was the picture of innocence in a country beaten down, and robbed, by a military regime happy to enrich itself while its citizens suffered.

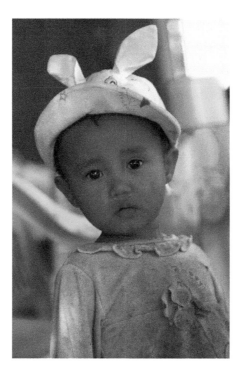

On December 26, 2004, a stretch of the deep Indian Ocean seabed some 600 miles long ruptured with the force of 23,000 Hiroshima-type atomic bombs, a 9.0-magnitude earthquake so powerful that it shifted the Earth's axis. Tsunamis smashed coastlines across the region, wreaking panic and catastrophe in 11 countries. Within hours, more than 150,000 people were dead or missing, and millions more had no homes. That morning, before the Earth shook with such vengeance, 3-year-old Sitalakshmi's mother tried to soothe a fussy, crying infant the way she often did, by giving the girl a grimy 10-rupee bill, worth about 25 cents at the time. When Sitalakshmi's big brown eyes caught mine, as she stared forlornly out the doorway of an Indian island orphanage not far from the quake's epicenter, she still squeezed the folded banknote tightly in her small fist. The girl wouldn't let go of it—even when she slept, a nun from Mother Teresa's Missionaries of Charity told me. Sitalakshmi was holding on to the memory of a mother, father and three brothers swept away when the tsunami hammered its first target: the Andaman and Nicobar Islands. The girl was alive because, when the ground began to violently shake, her brother, 14-year-old Balamurugan Kannan, bravely snatched her up and ran to higher ground fast enough to escape a wall of water rushing toward shore with the speed of a jet plane.

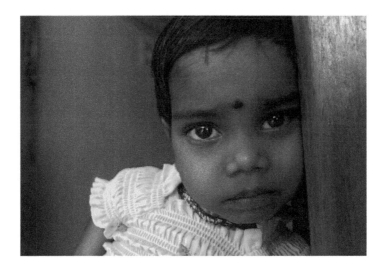

During the war in neighboring Vietnam, U.S. warplanes led by massive B-52 bombers flew more than half a million missions over Laos. They dropped between 2 and 3 million tons of bombs on Laos, which had a population of 3 million people. It was a ruthless attempt to deny Viet Cong guerrillas sanctuary. Long after they won, and the U.S. retreated from Vietnam in 1975, Laotians were still dying from unexploded ordinance, known to experts as UXO. The bombs lay in wait, often just below the muddy surface in the jungle, for decades before detonating. Several villagers, sitting

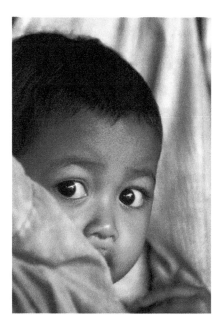

on the wooden floor of a village house in Makkheua, were telling me about the still lethal legacy of American bombing along the nearby Ho Chi Minh trail, when a child poked its head out, shyly trying to catch a glimpse of the strange visitor with the frightening questions on August 2, 2007. Over the previous three decades, the grisly toll from accidents involving UXO was 21 dead, 17 injured. Forty percent of the victims were children. I wondered whether the cute child playing eye tag with me would survive long enough to be safe from a war that was already history.

For decades, scientists have warned that warming seas would fuel bigger storms, which would kill many of the people who live along the world's shores. More powerful, and deadly, storms are just one of the dire consequences predicted from climate change. Cyclone Nargis may be a harbinger of worse to come. The hurricane, with winds exceeding 190 kilometers per hour, took aim at Myanmar's vulnerable underbelly, the central lowlands where a storm surge from the ocean flooded vast areas. More than 128,000 people died. The ruling junta didn't want embarrassing news coverage. I illegally hired a fishing boat, and lived on it as it moved through the worst-hit areas of the Irrawaddy River delta. For weeks, as poor farmers tried to survive in the ruins of homes that looked like they had exploded under the force of the winds, the generals in charge blocked most foreign relief aid. Chugging through the delta's maze of waterways, the fishing boat's pilot working the rusty tiller with his foot from the roof of the cabin where I worked, we came across corpses at practically every turn. After days lying in the water, tangled up in piles of broken trees and other debris, the only thing discernible about the dead were their clothes. The injured had to treat themselves. A traditional doctor splinted one man's broken arm with school rulers wrapped with filthy gauze. He salved the festering leg wound of another with a concoction made from mashed leaves. I reached the village of Kyaiktaw on May 11, 2008, where I photographed a girl so hungry that she sucked on her hand. Diarrhea was sapping what little strength she, and most other kids in the village, had left as they waited for help.

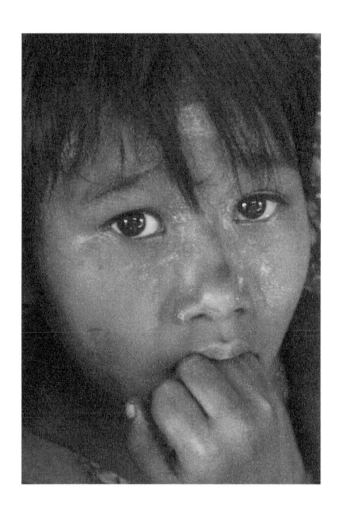

Knowing the U.S.-led war to oust Iraqi President Sadaam Hussein would soon reach their northern village, more than 150 Kurdish refugees fled and took shelter on a muddy hillside in seven trucks and ten, low-ceilinged tents made of tarps. For two days and nights before I reached their camp on March 26, 2003, howling wind and driving rain battered and clawed the flimsy plastic walls of their homes. The Kurds have a name for such relentless storms, which turn the sky an ominous black: the *rashaba*. Adults knew this one would pass, that as long as they could keep repairing tears in their tents, and keep the wind from shredding them, the sun would come again. But the children were terrified. For all they knew, the war they were trying to escape was now upon them. At night, it was near freezing. The kids were shoeless, and with only a kerosene stove and their own body heat to warm them, they were constantly cold. One family was huddled in a tent of blue plastic, which they had picked up in the local bazaar in the rush to open land. The tarp cast a frigid light over a girl standing at the partially opened flap. Her little brother lay in a wooden cradle just behind her, sucking on a pacifier, eyes fixed on me as I poked my head into their dank home. The girl froze, fighting back fresh tears. The storm wasn't so frightening anymore. The stooping stranger was something new to fear.

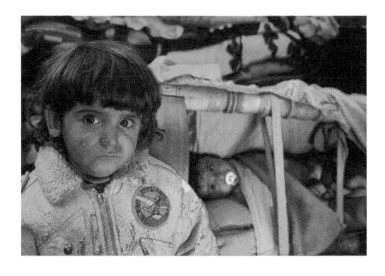

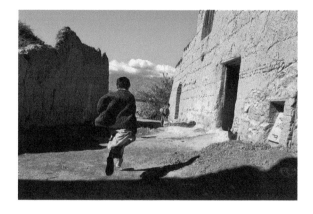

The Shomali Plain, the flatlands green with vineyards beneath towering mountains north of Kabul, has long held a special place in my mind. It was there, when years of war had destroyed the vineyards, and hoodoos of brown dust swirled like ghosts through empty villages, that I first saw the frontline. It was winter 1996, weeks after the Taliban had stormed into the capital, and Northern Alliance forces were on the run. I wanted to catch up with the legendary guerrilla leader Ahmad Shah Massoud, the warrior-intellectual who had held out against the Soviets in the rugged Panjshir Valley and was now fighting to hold back the Taliban. They were surprisingly accommodating to me. As volleys of rockets twice as long as my hired Volga soared from launchers on the plain, Talibs manning checkpoints waved me through with few questions. I was heading north to cross into no man's land and Massoud territory, but assured the Talibs that I only wanted to see the destruction Massoud had wrought before returning to my hotel in Kabul. On September 9, 2001, Al Qaeda killers posing as TV journalists assassinated Massoud with a suicide bomb blast, setting the stage for the attacks on the U.S. two days later. On October 6, 2003, I was back on the Shomali again, visiting the village Gala-e-Faiz. Saifullah Jan told me how the Taliban had forced his father out of their mudbrick home, murdered him and then set fire to the buildings and crops in 1996. As I left, a boy ran in front down a dirt path, almost floating on the freedom. The feeling was infectious. Maybe Afghans will finally have peace, I thought. Not even close.

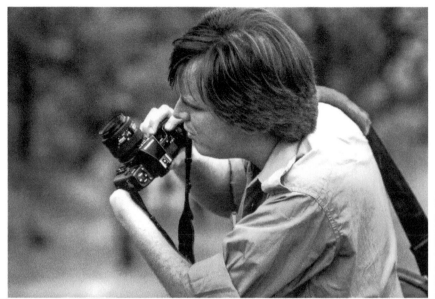

PHOTO BY: ANDREW STAWICKI

**Paul Watson** is a Canadian photojournalist. He was awarded the 1994 Pulitzer Prize for Spot News Photography for his photograph of U.S. Army Staff Sgt. William Cleveland's body being dragged by Somalis through the streets of Mogadishu. He is the author of three books: *Where War Lives*, *Magnum Revolution: 65 Years of Fighting for Freedom*, and *Ice Ghosts: The Epic Hunt for the Lost Franklin Expedition*. He is the subject of the Kennedy Award-winning play by Dan O'Brien entitled *The Body of an American*, which won the 2014 Horton Foote Prize for excellence in American theater and the PEN USA award for drama in 2013. His reporting and photography spans almost three decades and includes conflicts in Eritrea, Somalia, southern Sudan, Angola, Mozambique, South Africa, Romania, Serbia and Kosovo, Afghanistan, Pakistan, Kashmir, Iraq and Syria. While at the *Toronto Star*, Watson won four Canadian National Newspaper Awards for photography and stories on the child sex trade in Asia, anarchy in Somalia following the 1991 overthrow of dictator Mohammed Siad Barre, and the torture and murder of a Somali teen by Canadian soldiers after a U.S.-led force intervened to end a famine in 1992. His official website is arcticstarcreativity.com.

Alyssa

# It's Okay
# To Not
# Be Okay

Wooster

It started at 13, well at least my personal struggles did.

I had always been a bit chubby in elementary school, or as people so endearingly referred to it: having a "Buddha Belly" (which I still, to this day, hear as "boot-a-belly"). In high school I decided that I didn't want to have this "cute little baby fat" anymore. It started with sports. I danced, I played rugby, I played softball, I trained, I ran 5 Ks almost daily. I was exercising for hours on end. With the training of course I had to "fuel" my body, so then came the salads, the mere apple, all the good foods. Then came the growth—being my full 5'6" it was normal to be skinny after a growth spurt, right?

First 100 pounds, then 90 pounds, then 80. I was ranging around a BMI of 13.7, but I was just growing, right? My family was worried, but I wasn't. A friend approached me saying maybe I shouldn't go for another run, being the first one to call me the big "A" word. I was skinny, I was "beautiful" in my own mind. I couldn't control the acne, or the braces, or the bangs (another regrettable choice at that age), but my weight—well I could control that.

I didn't realize that I was struggling with anorexia until years later (like many of my other struggles). Luckily, I got better. I had put on (the minimal) amount of weight to be acceptable. My aunt stopped worrying, my friends stopped commenting. Growing up in a dance studio and working at a restaurant known to hire people for their looks, I grew up hating my body, I hated myself, I hated my appearance, but most of all I hated my mind.

I wish I could say that that was the extent of my struggle with mental illness, but unfortunately it was just the first shovelful from the pit I would later fall into. If you asked anyone who knew me in high school, they would describe me as a good student, a girl who occasionally liked to party, an active individual, and a really nice, happy girl! Working, volunteering, dancing and having straight A's was my way of distracting myself from myself. If I studied a bit longer for this test, I wouldn't have to worry about lying in my bed until 4 in the morning thinking about all the horrible things I had done, and the horrible things I wish I could do.

The deep dark depression consumed me. I masked it with a smile and took part in all sorts of activities.

Grade 11 was the first diagnoses—Major Depressive Disorder—it felt like a stamp on my forehead that everyone could see. My therapist suggested medication, but I refused to admit that I couldn't function like everyone else. I didn't need it, and going on medication seemed like giving up on any hope of being "normal." So I spent no time alone, leaving myself no time to think. Immersing myself in activities, before my depression drowned me.

Then began the anxiety, dancing with the depression. I had been asked to join the professional division of my dance studio for Hip Hop—to be alongside the best dancers at the studio, who I admired and placed on a pedestal. I did not feel worthy of being at this level. My feelings of inadequacy, in the one field I had always felt good at, overwhelmed me.

That was the year I started having my "asthma attacks." They soon came more often. Would I get accepted into McGill? Queen's? How did I only get a 90? The words *failure failure failure* ate at me until I couldn't breathe, I couldn't think. I sat in a puddle of tears and anxiety, begging to catch my breath. It wasn't until after being diagnosed with a Generalized Anxiety Disorder two years later—Panic subtype—that I realized they were not asthma attacks. I pushed myself through my depression and anxiety. I told myself that life at university will be better. It'll be better, I'll be happy. It was the Holy Land to me.

McGill, I had made it, the top university in Canada. Life had to be better there. It was as if I could leave my mental illnesses back in Vancouver: apparently I believed that they wouldn't be able to get through the airport security at YVR, but unfortunately I was wrong.

Residence seemed like it would be the best time of my life. A new start, new friends, away from the toxicity of my old life at home. But there were things I didn't expect, the change in course load, being constantly surrounded by people. I went from having a 94% average to barely getting B's. My anxiety would make my mind blank. I would sit in exams shaking, unable to concentrate, just trying to take a deep breath, trying to not let myself go into a full-blown panic attack and embarrass myself in a field-house full of people.

I didn't expect the partying. I didn't think I would ever have a bad relationship with alcohol, having a family member who struggles with addiction. I was careful, diligent. But I found that harder to control. I would drink until I no longer felt anxious and often would drink to the point of becoming unaware of my actions. Blacking out. This sent me into an horrible anxiety-inducing cycle of waking up in the morning having no recollection of what had happened the night before, panicking as I had no idea how I had gotten home, who I had talked to, or where I had been. But that was university, right? We all party a bit too hard. I thought the panic would stop in university, but it didn't. It was all consuming. I was a failure, I was worthless. How can I not handle the course load? I used to be such a good student.

My anxiety got in the way of new friendships. My friends thought I was upset with them as I would lock myself in my room, to keep the panic contained within my four small dorm room walls. And it kept getting worse. I would take the back stairs to avoid talking to anyone. But it was just school. That's why I would hide from my friends, my emotions. Myself.

I struggled with not falling back into my ED (eating disorder) tendencies, after the freshman 15 came (and went) and the stress consumed me. Then school stopped, but the anxiety didn't. I spent the first 18 years of my life trying to run away from the truth, giving myself set points: when you make it here you'll be better, when you get here you'll be happy. It didn't.

You're smart, you're strong, you can beat this. But I couldn't and I can't on my own. That's why I finally made the decision to go on medication. Anti-depressants were horrifying to me. Everyone has a bit of anxiety, but after my first month of medication, I realized I hadn't been functioning at a normal level. I was overwhelmed by the ability to stay calm. It was jarring. I didn't realize that not every 18-year-old felt my constant state of worrying and ruminating and panicking.

Going on medication was the best and most difficult decision I've ever made. Years of therapy have helped, but there's a point in your life where you can no longer let other people help you. You need to help yourself. I remember sitting in my doctor's office, the woman I had seen as a child, describing to her that I couldn't be rational, I couldn't be around people, I couldn't feel normal. She was the second person to ever suggest I go on medication and this time I accepted. I finally admitted that I couldn't do this alone. It wasn't simply an issue of willpower, it was a mental illness.

When friends express worries about their mental health to me, I am quick to console, I tell them that anxiety and depression are diseases of chemicals not characters, but this is a phrase I struggle with daily. And chemicals can be regulated. A friend once said to me: medication doesn't stop the waves, it just gives you a board and a paddle. Sometimes it can be hard to admit you can't swim.

My panic attacks have calmed down. It's rare that my anxiety consumes me fully. Well, at least it's less often than it used to be, and I feel like I (for the most part) have a better relationship with food now. I'm not 100 percent happy, nor do I think I ever will be. I know that it is a constant struggle, that I can never eat anything without thinking twice, and there's rarely a day that goes by without some sadness. But that's part of living with a mental illness. You may not ever be 100 percent okay, but it's also okay to not be okay.

I struggle with not knowing when I will feel okay, but I have the resources and strength to deal with my emotions until I do.

———

**Alyssa Wooster** is a recent graduate in psychology from McGill University. She spent her time there doing research and front-line work in harm reduction. She currently lives in Montreal. She hopes to pursue her master's degree in Public Health in the upcoming years, working to make the public mental health sector more accessible. When she is not working, she enjoys reading, cooking, and catching up on what's new on Netflix. An earlier draft of this piece was written at age 19 and originally published on ProjectPilgrim.org. Alyssa is now 23 years old.

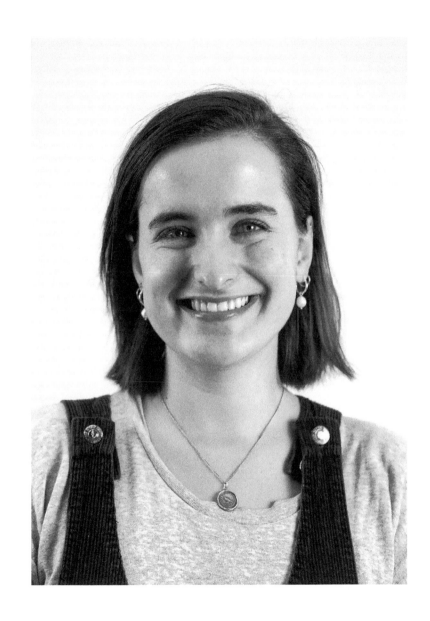

Bänoo

# The Mirror
# Soliloquy

Zan

I.

Here I am
and Evin is far away

I've been its inmate in dreams
Its gates open to secrets

The sentence of life—
the interrogation of regret—
Good-bye is the kindest exit here

It is an honour—
known for its unknown

the prison of fear
I never broke out of
fearing the death I was going through

You, fellow-inmate borders away,
There is no air
as I sabotage your solitary cell

Paint the walls with
your hunger
Strike the food-fed in the face

Your bones are broken
unlike the beast I am

Every revolution hijacks treason
The tongue of truth is a swollen tell-tale

I revel in paralysis—

proud of disgust and—
dead


II.

What is the genre of pain?

I cannot translate it into a story
Chronology kills it in the beginning, middle and end

Time strips teasingly out of truth
Its contours curve
sensual, sadistic, serene

Desire thrusts itself into exile
and I moan out of myself

I cannot write me
I'm not what I write
I'm the writer who writes me

My paper stains
the dark


III.

This is the prophecy of breakout
There is nowhere but you

and the pain loves you so much
you cannot leave

and you love it so much
you cannot forget

You need it
to go through yourself

Let the serpent
bite its tale

It's blood you need
to be more than you are

Distance
travels in your journey
and brings you home


IV.

Green is not the colour of ink
Make yourself legible

Visit pain—
your forbidden love—
as windows wonder at the world

Bend
your ribs

Don't sell politics
for a poultice

You are not a sleep—
You are a dream

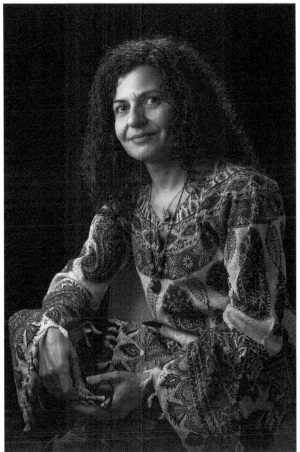

PHOTO BY: ALEX USQUIANO

**Bänoo Zan** is a poet, librettist, translator, teacher, editor, and poetry curator with numerous published poems as well as three books. *Song of Phoenix: Life and Works of Sylvia Plat*h, was published in Iran. *Songs of Exile*, published by Guernica Editions—and where this poem first appeared—was shortlisted for the Gerald Lampert Memorial Award by the League of Canadian Poets. *Letters to My Father* was published by Piquant Press. She founded Shab-e She'r, Toronto's most diverse poetry open mic series, in 2012. It bridges the gap between ethnicities, nationalities, religions (or lack thereof), ages, genders, sexual orientations, disabilities, poetic styles, voices and visions.

# Acknowledgements

——

As the editors, we have been inspired by the honesty of the words and the images gathered within *A Perfect Offering*, we have been humbled by the willingness of all contributors to share their heart-holding stories, and we are honoured to include them in this book.

We would also like to thank the following for their support and for connecting us to contributors we would not otherwise have contacted: Julie Albert, Lida Alirezaei, John Armstrong, Christie Blatchford, Peter Bogdanovich, Michele Coleman, Mike Downie, Robert Everett-Green, Charlotte Forbes, Camilla Gibb, Mary Jo Haddad, Chaviva Hošek, Tim Huggins, Ania Idzik, Lucy Kalanithi, David Kinahan, David Leonard, Seblé Makonnen, Tulu Makonnen, Jennifer Meeropol, Robert Meeropol, David Mitchell, Walter Mosley, Sheilagh O'Connell, Siobhan O'Connell, Elana Rabinovitch, Rita M. Reichart, Julia Rhodes, Bob Shantz, Adam Sol, Andrew Taylor, Andrea Wojnicki, and Morden Yolles.

Thanks to our agent Michael Levine—in a tough market, he has always been interested in this book and its intents. And a special thanks to Howard Aster of Mosaic Press for his early, steadfast, and continuing devotion to this project. Howard is also responsible for securing the graphic expertise of Andrea Tempesta, who has helped shape the look and feel of the book with his compelling and sympathetic design.

**Harold Heft** wrote three books, including *The Shape of This Dying: Remembering Alexander Bercovitch* (Mosaic) and *Build a Better Book Club* (Macmillan Canada, written with Peter O'Brien). For many years, he published articles and reviews in *The Globe and Mail, National Post, The Jewish Daily Forward, Montreal Gazette and Tablet.* A graduate of McGill University, and with a PhD in literature from the University of Western Ontario, he taught both English and film there, and was a visiting fellow at The Hebrew University of Jerusalem. He worked as a senior strategist and marketing communications executive at various universities and hospitals, including the University of Toronto where he met his wife, Suzanne, at North York General Hospital, and at The Hospital for Sick Children. At age 51, after a diagnosis of an inoperable brain tumour, and after a heroic fight to prolong his life, Harold died on 23 July 2015.

**Suzanne Heft** was born in Nova Scotia to an American father and an Iraqi mother. She grew up in the U.S., the Middle East and Europe, with her head bent over a book, riveted by stories, especially those of redemption and transformation. As a student at the University of Toronto, she studied English literature, and after a stint working in public relations, she became a passionate advocate for worthy charitable causes as a fundraising executive. She has worked to build organizational capacity and philanthropic investment in some of Canada's most prominent secondary and post-secondary institutions, including her *alma mater*, the University of Toronto. She still looks for powerful stories every day, in books and in the world. She is the mother of two teenage sons and the wife of Harold Heft.

**Peter O'Brien** has written or edited seven books, including *Introduction to Literature: British, American, Canadian* (Harper & Row), *Build a Better Book Club* (Macmillan Canada, written with Harold Heft), and *Cleopatra at the Breakfast Table: Why I Studied Latin With My Teenager and How I Discovered the Daughterland* (Quattro). Born in New York, he has a BA from Notre Dame, an MA from McGill, and he attended the Banff School of Fine Arts. He has nine brothers and sisters, and 12 step-brothers and -sisters. He has published articles and reviews in *The Globe and Mail, Toronto Star* and *Montreal Gazette*. He has worked as a shoe salesman, a roughneck on oil rigs, a fundraiser, an environmental entrepreneur, and in corporate communications. He was a founding Board member of White Ribbon, the world's largest movement of men and boys working to end violence against women and girls. He exhibits and publishes his artwork LOTS OF FUN WITH FINNEGANS WAKE internationally.

**A Perfect Offering**
Personal stories of trauma and transformation